M000159215

MICROSCOPY HANDBOOKS 31

# Scientific PhotoMACROgraphy

# Royal Microscopical Society MICROSCOPY HANDBOOKS

# Scientific PhotoMACROgraphy

**Brian Bracegirdle**

Cold Aston Lodge, Cold Aston, Cheltenham, Glos. GL54 3BN, UK

In association with the Royal Microscopical Society

© **Brian Bracegirdle, 1995**

Brian Bracegirdle has asserted his right to be identified as the author of this work in accordance with the Copyright, Designs and Patents Act 1988.

First published 1995

A CIP catalogue for this book is available from the British Library.

ISBN 1 872748 49 X

**BIOS Scientific Publishers Ltd**
**St Thomas House, Becket Street, Oxford, OX1 1SJ, UK**
**Tel. +44 (0) 1865 726286. Fax. +44 (0) 1865 246823**

DISTRIBUTORS

*Australia and New Zealand*
  DA Information Services
  648 Whitehorse Road, Mitcham
  Victoria 3132

*Singapore and South East Asia*
  Toppan Company (S) PTE Ltd
  38 Liu Fang Road, Jurong
  Singapore 2262

*India*
  Viva Books Private Limited
  4346/4C Ansari Road
  New Delhi 110002

*USA and Canada*
  Books International Inc.
  PO Box 605, Herndon, VA 22070

Typeset by AMA Graphics Ltd, Preston, UK.
Printed by The Alden Press Ltd, Oxford, UK.

# Contents

# Abbreviations

| | |
|---|---|
| CCD | charge-coupled device |
| CCTV | closed circuit television |
| DIC | differential interference contrast |
| NA | numerical aperture |
| OTF | off-the-film |
| RC | resin-coated |
| RMS | Royal Microscopical Society |
| TTL | through-the-lens |
| WORM | write once, read many |

# Preface

In the past, making photographs of microscopical preparations and other objects in the range between about × 1 and about × 50 has been difficult to achieve with high quality. A large range of equipment, *ad hoc* and purpose-made, has been described and offered, and much has been written on technique. With modern apparatus and materials, such records are much easier to obtain, but the correct procedure is vital if disappointment is to be avoided. This book considers only more modern equipment, and thus omits much that would nowadays be merely tedious, such as a consideration of obsolete methods of estimating exposure.

Quite different approaches are needed for transmitted-light work and reflected-light work, and this is mirrored in the arrangement of the book. This concentrates on *technique*, and uses many illustrations of apparatus, partly for direct instruction in how to set them up, and partly to act as inspiration for designing and modifying one's own equipment. One of the most important parts of a laboratory specializing in close-range work is a basic workshop! Photographs of the *results* of the work are rarely included; they often need colour plates to do them justice, and many examples are already available elsewhere.

It is a pleasure to acknowledge the encouragement and help received from my friend and colleague of many years, Savile Bradbury. His advice on the first draft was, as ever, cogent and concise; as editor of the series he brings great enthusiasm and industry to bear, not least on his authors. Similarly, in our publishers we have a company who, refreshingly, produce a good-quality book from a manuscript in record time and with great efficiency.

The fruits of 30 years of involvement in photomacrography are offered in this book, in the hope that readers will find their frustration minimized and results of quality easier to obtain.

Brian Bracegirdle
Cheltenham, 1994

xi

# Safety

Attention to safety aspects is an integral part of all laboratory procedures and both the Health and Safety at Work Act and the COSHH regulations impose legal requirements on those persons planning or carrying out such procedures.

In this and other Handbooks every effort has been made to ensure that the recipes, formulae and practical procedures are accurate and safe. However, it remains the responsibility of the reader to ensure that the procedures which are followed are carried out in a safe manner and that all necessary COSHH requirements have been looked up and implemented. Any specific safety instructions relating to items of laboratory equipment must also be followed.

# 1 The Scope of the Process

The production of images magnified in the range $\times 1$ to $\times 50$ is the traditional preserve of photomacrography. Below $\times 1$ ordinary photographic equipment can be used to make close-up photographs, and above $\times 50$ the compound microscope is used to make photomicrographs. Why this distinction, and why a special book? It is a matter, in this range of magnifications, of very specialized techniques and equipment.

On the one hand, close-ups of a fair quality can be made (as can photographs at infinity) with many ordinary cameras, even hand-held ones. The object in such cases is not too small to handle easily nor too small to illuminate easily, and it may even be pictured using available light. On the other hand, with the compound microscope, although much superfluous material has been written in the past on photomicrography (but see Bradbury, 1989; Richardson, 1991; Thomson and Bradbury, 1987) especially before modern equipment was available, and especially by those who preferred designing and making up equipment to using it, both lighting and specimen support do tend to be standardized in modern equipment. Thus, the process of using the microscope to make an image for recording is simpler, while cameras can often very easily be attached if they are not actually built-in.

## 1.1 The macro range

The macro range, in between these two extremes, has always tended to be a more difficult area to work in. Classically, a lens of relatively short focal length was used on a generally horizontal camera at a long extension to produce a magnified image. This gave rise to all manner of difficulties (as will be described), and a wide range of equipment. Older equipment will not be described here if it is no longer useful; it belongs to the history of photomacrography, which has already been summarized elsewhere (Bracegirdle, 1982). Some other sources on macro-range work include Bracegirdle (1983), Lefkowitz (1979), Loveland (1970) and White (1987). Illustrations of results are to be found in Thompson *et al*. (1981) and Anon. (1977).

1

Nowadays, in addition to updated (usually vertical) apparatus using one lens at long extension (*Figure 1.1*), images in the macro range are often generated by compound systems, some of them specially manufactured for use at these magnifications; therefore, the old definition of macro work (using one lens only) is no longer tenable. In addition to these specialist zoom macro units (such as the excellent M400 PhotoMakroskop series by Wild and the earlier Tessovar by Zeiss), simple tubular adapters are commonplace, which allow one tube of stereomicroscopes to be used to make photographs at macro magnifications, or which can be used as more complicated trinocular adapters for simultaneous viewing and recording.

The precise means adopted to secure the required magnification will be discussed below, but several general difficulties apply however the desired magnification is obtained.

## 1.2 General difficulties

General difficulties are: (i) limited depth of field, (ii) the deleterious effects of vibration, and (iii) difficulties in accurate focusing; all are endemic in the macro range. Difficulties in illumination are different according to whether transmitted or reflected lighting is used, and will therefore be discussed in the appropriate separate chapters, as will exposure estimation. Difficulties in exposure estimation are largely obviated with modern equipment, but will be mentioned in the contexts of calibration and of temporary set-ups.

### 1.2.1 Depth of field

Depth of field is determined by two factors, regardless of the means by which the image is obtained (a fuller treatment is given by Clarke, 1984). One is the effective aperture, the other is the magnification. Although some modern television-based instruments appear to avoid this limitation of physical optics, by providing a large depth of field at high magnification, in fact they all make up their apparently static image from a number of scans of a beam, the image being formed relatively slowly from several different levels. This suffices for many purposes, although the quality obtained is far from that of a photographic film. It is often depressing to have to accept that in all systems forming an image not derived from scanning, the two factors already mentioned, and they alone, always operate. The equation for depth of field is:

$$2cf(m+1)/m^2,$$

where $c$ = the diameter of the maximum acceptable circle of confusion, $f$ = the *effective f* number, and m = magnification.

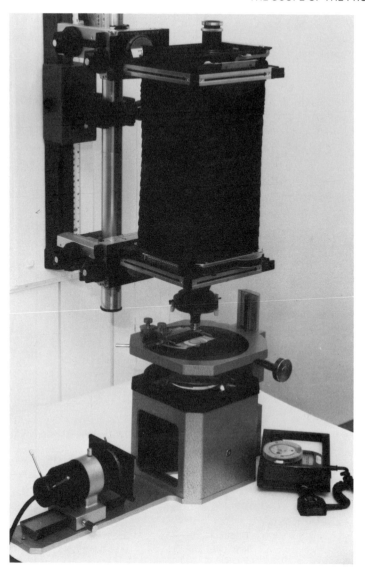

**Figure 1.1:** Modern vertical photomacrographic bench.

The Nikon Multiphot macro-dia base is supported on a heavy levelling table 300 mm above floor level. A decentrable iris diaphragm and long lamp-centring screws have been added to the unit, and the frosted glass has been removed from the collector-lens train. The camera is a $4 \times 5$ inch Sinar P, with extra rails added, so that wherever the lens and rear standards are sited, they are fully supported. It carries the Sinar shutter (with a very wide opening and range of speeds B, 1/60 – 1, 2, 3, 4, 6, 8 sec) as well as a Compur Electronic 1 shutter (which works totally without vibration and has speeds 1/500 – 32 sec + T), shown carried on a snout. The focusing screen has a coverglass cemented at its centre, over a pencilled cross, and the separate $\times 8$ lens is focused on the cross to allow parallax-free focusing at low magnifications. The two rail clamps carrying the Sinar are attached to long carriers sliding and clamping anywhere along the length of a 1 m, student-type, triangular-section optical bench, bolted truly vertically to the wall, with a scale alongside. This allows total flexibility in positioning the camera vertically, while ensuring that it is rigid at all times. The movements of the camera are available for setting up, and for use in reflected-light work.

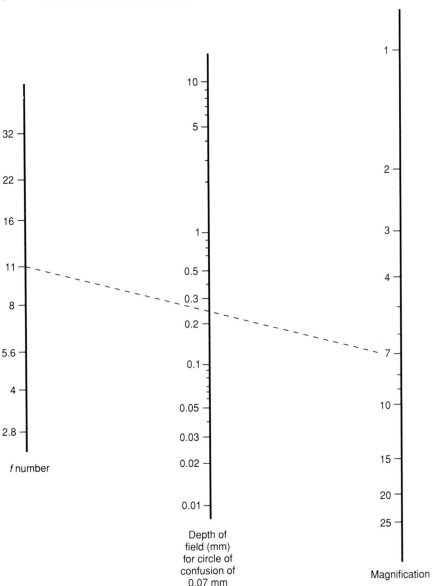

**Figure 1.2:**   Depth of field nomogram.

The accompanying depth of field nomogram (*Figure 1.2*) provides a convenient summary for a circle of confusion (see opposite) suitable for much photographic work, and demonstrates that at magnifications of only about × 10, a depth of field of 0.5 mm is a luxury. If all else fails, it is possible to increase this by making a photograph of a small object at a smaller magnification than is finally needed, and then enlarging the resulting negative to a greater extent than normal. It has to be remembered that one is then merely making an enlargement of a dispersion of particles of silver or of pigment, and not of the original object; final resolution is lower and noise is magnified. For reflected-light work, apparent depth of field can be increased by using a sheet of light and winding up the (suitably shaped) object through it, as described in Chapter 4. For transmitted-light work, even the small depth of field normally obtained is almost always adequate for the permanent preparations usually being recorded.

## 1.2.2 Circle of confusion

The permitted circle of confusion at the focal plane requires some further consideration. No optical system produces a point image of a point object – the image is always a circle (called a circle of confusion or antipoint). This circle can be tiny (if the system is highly corrected and the object is accurately in focus), or larger (if the system is less well corrected and the object is not accurately in focus). It gets larger as the focus worsens, thus giving rise to the concept of depth of field, the limits of lens-to-subject distance outside which sharpness is unacceptable. The average human eye cannot see detail finer than 0.075 mm, and thus there is no need to have points rendered smaller than this diameter in the picture *at its final magnification*. Points rendered at a diameter of 0.25 mm or larger are unacceptable to the average eye. For practical purposes, it is possible to summarize the apertures required at various magnifications (for a circle of confusion of 0.075 mm) as given in *Table 1.1*.

**Table 1.1:**   Numerical apertures (NAs) required at various magnifications

| Magnification on negative | NA required | Equivalent $f$ number |
|---|---|---|
| × 1 | 0.003 | $f$ 75 |
| × 2 | 0.007 | $f$ 50 |
| × 3 | 0.010 | $f$ 38 |
| × 5 | 0.017 | $f$ 25 |
| × 10 | 0.033 | $f$ 14 |
| × 20 | 0.067 | $f$ 7 |
| × 30 | 0.100 | $f$ 5 |
| × 40 | 0.135 | $f$ 3.5 |
| × 50 | 0.167 | $f$ 3 |

However, some macro lenses are not marked with $f$ numbers, but with an arbitrary series indicating the increase in exposure required. Furthermore, as the size of the negative increases (thus allowing smaller enlargement to a standard final print size), larger circles of confusion are allowable. A nomogram to accommodate these variables has in practice proved entirely workable for many years (see *Figure 1.3*).

## 1.2.3 Susceptibility to vibration

Susceptibility to vibration was an especial consequence of using traditional horizontal long-bellows equipment, but also affects some other

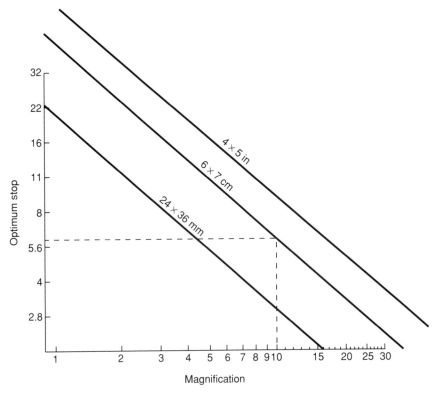

**Figure 1.3:** Optimum-stop nomogram.
'Optimum stop' gives the maximum depth of field consistent with no loss of general sharpness due to diffraction. Calculated for permissible circles of confusion: 24 × 36 mm – 0.03 mm; 6 × 7 cm – 0.07 mm; 4 × 5 inch – 0.1 mm.

apparatus. Whereas a compound microscope is compact, with its centre of gravity low-placed when the camera is vertically above it for photomicrography, a long horizontal set-up is made to vibrate only too easily, and this becomes very obvious at higher magnifications. In this regard, it cannot be too highly stressed that it is hardly possible to support macro equipment on too massive a stand. Those using macro-range photography professionally on a daily basis, to record living organisms in studio aquaria or to make eye-level views of science-fiction model sets for television against deadlines, have their equipment supported on several H-section, rolled-steel joists of section at least 8 inches, embedded in solid concrete, and with massive crossmembers welded in place (*Figure 1.4*). For those making a permanent set-up for macro work, this approach, or a modification of it, has everything to commend it, if space and funds allow. If not, every effort should still be made to make the base of the equipment heavy, with supports bolted into place. For example, standard (new) steel scaffolding poles are inexpensive, easily and very firmly joined by the clips used in normal erection at building sites, and provide a solid base for mounting other equipment to them. Once initial lining-up has been achieved, such

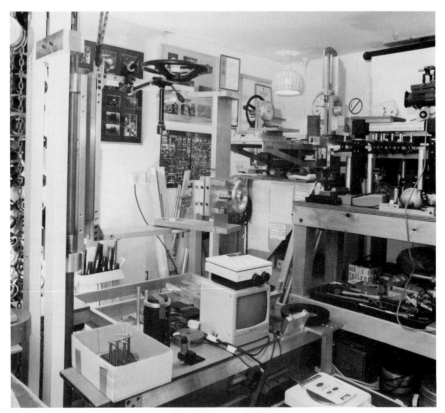

**Figure 1.4:** Heavy supports for professional motion-picture work.

In the foreground a partly-assembled vertical optical bench has a camera support platform (capable of carrying two IMAX cameras, each incorporating 14 servomotors, of total weight 250 kg, for stereo filming), which can be rotated through 360° using the large handwheel on top. The bench below has motor-driven movement in all three axes, and carries a rotating table able to support 500 kg. In the background, below the other handwheel, is a bench built up from heavy tube sections secured to wall and floor; in front of this a heavy platform sits on very heavy brackets, to carry the same cameras. The ends of the rolled steel joists carrying the platform are sunk into concrete. The horizontal bench in front carries the subjects up to 2 tonnes in weight (often small living organisms in aquaria, but rigged as required) on highly mobile motor-driven platforms. Total rigidity is the requirement when 1000 ft of film is used every 3 min, at magnifications up to × 250 as routine. All parts are mounted on linear or circular roller bearings, all are motorized, and all sections of metal used in the purpose-made constructions are extra heavy. Photograph made by kind permission of Peter Parks, Image Quest 3D Ltd.

an apparatus will obviate difficulties arising from lack of rigidity, and will also allow equipment to be attached to it on secure anti-vibration mounts. Specialist commercial companies supply a range of modern and very effective anti-vibration mounts, and some more general suppliers such as Electromail, the retail mail order division of RS Components (see Appendix) also carry a useful range. Such devices are easily available, inexpensive, and some can act in any attitude. The traditional method of providing vibration damping for a horizontal arrangement was to put three rubber balls into a piece of heavy ceramic sewage pipe, 2 inches long and 6 inches in diameter, with a fourth resting in the depression between the first three balls to accept the (horizontal) load. Several of these under a platform will damp vibrations very effectively and cheaply, providing the balls are renewed about once a year. For modern vertical-axis equipment, heavy right-angle brackets attached to verticals such as the scaffolding tubing already mentioned will carry antivibration mounts, to which crossmembers are attached to carry the vertical rails; use of such parts will obviate even very pronounced vibrations.

## 1.2.4 Accuracy in focusing at low power

Focusing accurately can be a difficulty at lower magnifications, as the eye may accommodate (and focus on the image above or below the focal plane) unless prevented from doing so. For 35 mm cameras, a suitable (possibly waist-level type) viewfinder may be used, of the kind having a supplementary lens above the screen; a better alternative is a right-angle adapter (which incorporates a focusable magnifier), and another is a definite macro focuser. All these focus at the right level (on markings on the ground surface) and thus prevent the eye from registering an image not in the

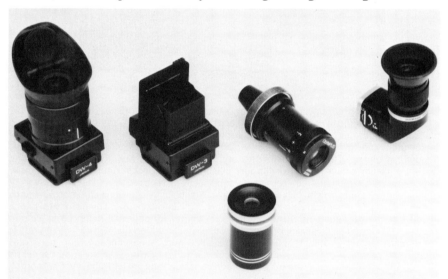

**Figure 1.5:** Finders and magnifiers for parallax-free focusing at low magnifications.
On the left is the focusing magnifying finder DW-4 (magnifying × 6) for the Nikon F3, and the waist-level DW-3 with pop-up × 5 lens next to it. To be able to interchange finders on a 35 mm camera is very helpful, and an important point in the choice of a camera body for macro and micro work; the screens must also be interchangeable, of course. Third from left is an attachable magnifier with graticule for the Olympus attachable shutter for microscope use. On the right is the Olympus attachable Varimagni × 1.2/× 2.5 focusable magnifying right-angle viewer, typical of such an attachment for a camera without interchangeable viewfinders. Below is an ordinary focusable × 8 magnifier, for use directly on a ground-glass screen of larger format (see *Figure 1.1*). At low magnifications it is difficult to prevent the eye accommodating slightly when viewing the image; this can be avoided only by using a magnifier focused on the image plane and by moving the eye slightly from side to side when using it to ensure that the image does not seem to move with it. If it does not move, the image is sharply focused in the plane of the screen.

plane of the screen as sharp (*Figure 1.5*). If the interchangeable screen itself is of the type which is plain-ground with a central clear window (unfortunately available only for more expensive cameras), this is an advantage. In any case, the usual cycle of slight lateral movements of the eye to check for focus by lack of parallax should always be employed. For larger formats, the ground-glass screen should always have a coverglass cemented to its centre, over a central fine pencilled cross on the ground surface (as is the norm for high-power work also). It is necessary always to use the usual $\times 8$ magnifier on the screen when setting focus; the magnifier must of course be precisely focused on the cross.

# References

**Anon.** (1977) *Close-up Photography and Photomacrography* (Eastman Kodak publication N–12). Rochester, NY.

**Bracegirdle B.** (1982) A history of photomacrography. *Proc. R. Microsc. Soc.*, **17**, 316–326.

**Bracegirdle B.** (1983) An outline of technique for photomacrography. *Proc. R. Microsc. Soc.*, **18**, 105–117.

**Bradbury S.** (1989) *An Introduction to the Optical Microscope*, revised edn (RMS Handbook 01). Oxford University Press, Oxford.

**Clarke TM.** (1984) Method for calculating relative apertures for optimizing diffraction-limited depth of field in photomacrography. *The Microscope*, **32**, 219–258.

**Lefkowitz L.** (1979) *The Manual of Close-up Photography*. Amphoto, Garden City.

**Loveland RP.** (1970) Low power photomicrography with transmitted light. In *Photomicrography: A Comprehensive Treatise*, vol. 1. Wiley, New York pp. 220–238.

**Richardson JH.** (1991) *Handbook for the Light Microscope*. Noyes, Park Ridge.

**Thomson DJ, Bradbury S.** (1987) *An Introduction to Photomicrography* (RMS Handbook 13). Oxford University Press, Oxford.

**Thompson G., Bernard G, Cooke J. et al.** (1981) *Focus on Nature*. Faber, London.

**White W. (ed.)** (1987) *Photomacrography: An Introduction*. Focal Press, London.

# 2 Obtaining the Magnification

## 2.1 Lens formulae

In the classical equipment, using a single lens to form an image, as the lens is moved further from the screen than its infinity position (i.e. its focal length) so the image is more and more highly magnified (*Figure 2.1*). The classic formulae relating focal length $(F)$ to object $(u)$ and image $(v)$ distances are:

$$1/F = 1/u + 1/v,$$
$$v = Fu/u - F$$

and

$$u = Fv/v - F.$$

Magnification (m) is given by:

$$m = F/u - F = v - F/F.$$

A much-used equation combining the two is that for bellows extension:

$$v = F(m + 1).$$

A handy nomogram providing this information directly is given in *Figure 2.2*.

When using the above equations, it should be borne in mind that all normal camera lenses are computed for use with the object distance as a much longer conjugate distance than the image distance, and that since these values are reversed once the image is the same size (at an extension equal to twice the focal length of the lens), normal lenses used normally reveal spherical aberration and provide soft images. Specially computed macro lenses are designed to have these conjugate distances normally reversed, and are thus suited to macro-range work, but not to standard photography.

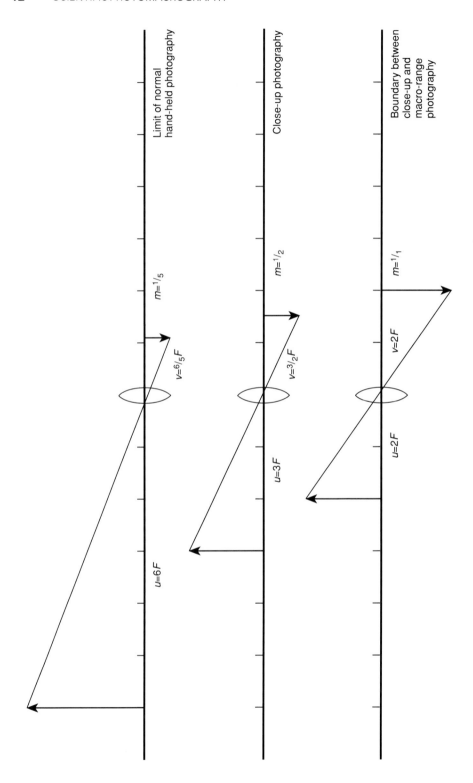

Limit of normal hand-held photography

$m=1/5$

$v=6/5 F$

$u=6F$

Close-up photography

$m=1/2$

$v=3/2 F$

$u=3F$

Boundary between close-up and macro-range photography

$m=1/1$

$v=2F$

$u=2F$

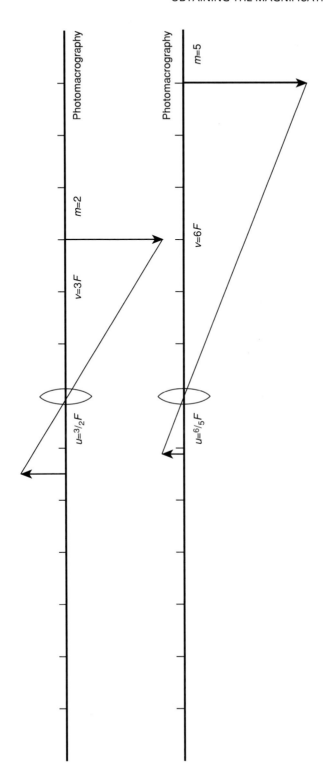

**Figure 2.1:** Object and image distances.
$F$, focal length of lens; $m$, magnification; $u$ object distance; $v$, image distance.

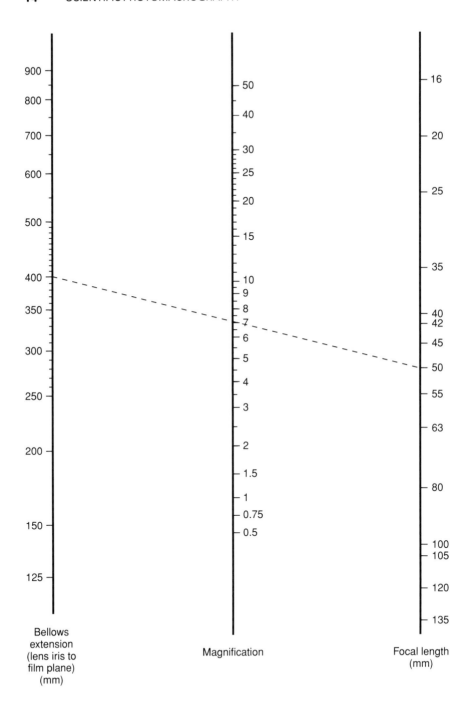

Bellows extension (lens iris to film plane) (mm)

Magnification

Focal length (mm)

**Figure 2.2:** Magnification nomogram.

## 2.2 The field of view required

The field of view required is, in practice, the usual controlling factor in selecting the lens and other equipment. If a specific magnification is to be set, this is usually done after the lens covering the field of view has been chosen. Given a choice, it is usually best practice to use the longest focal length which will give the required magnification; the working distance is greater, and in reflected-light work this is important, as it gives more space to arrange lighting and a better perspective.

It is a recommended exercise when setting up macro equipment for the first time, as part of the initial calibration work, to determine the fields of view delivered with transmitted light by the available lens and condenser combinations. If an England finder (Graticules Ltd, see Appendix) is used as the object, its ruled squares of side 1 mm not only provide a definite value for field diameter, but also act as a stage micrometer to determine magnification; they are also flat and give contrast to provide a test target for the assessment of image quality. The 1 mm spacings all over the surface of the standard $3 \times 1$ inch slide are ideal for these purposes at higher magnifications in the macro range, and possession of such a slide is highly desirable. For the lowest magnifications, a flat transparent rule graduated in millimetres and centimetres is suitable. For setting up and testing the lower powers, a sheet of dry lettering (such as Letraset) carrying a selection of circles of various sizes is excellent as an inexpensive test target. Such sheets are of high quality, with accurately sized and perfectly printed components, and pieces of them can be used with both transmitted and reflected illumination.

## 2.3 Setting and checking magnification

Setting and checking magnification is also best done with the England finder, after initial adjustments according to the above formulae or nomogram. If precise magnifications are required, they cannot usually be set by measuring distances, as it is not always possible to know where the nodal point of the lens is situated, even if its focal length is as engraved. With the finder, direct readings are obtained in the image plane, before the settings are locked, after which focusing is carried out by moving the whole camera, or the stage, with the object centred again. If very high ($> \times 35$) magnifications are arranged macroscopically, an ordinary stage micrometer may be used to check magnifications on the 0.1 mm rulings. Such stage micrometers are, of course, available in reflected-light versions also.

## 2.4 Suitable lenses

Suitable lenses that are not part of a purpose-built macroscope have been mentioned above as specially computed macro lenses. They are supplied by microscope (as opposed to camera) manufacturers, are of simple construction (with only a few elements in very few groups), and in the shorter focal lengths are normally in mounts with RMS threads. It has already been said that their longer conjugate distances are behind them, but this does not mean that they will give of their best at all magnifications. Each has a definite best magnification, and an acceptable range round this. In practice, this means that extremes of bellows length are to be avoided. Do not seek to attain high magnifications by using longer-focus lenses on very long bellows extensions.

In the past, many firms have offered such special macro lenses, and many are still available, perhaps in forgotten cupboards in departments, or perhaps on the secondhand market. The crucial difference between older and newer macro lenses, apart from any advances in computation and the use of new optical glasses, is that the new ones are coated or multi-coated. This is a most important difference in obtaining a crisp image. Do not use old macro lenses if you seek good results!

Recently, a variety of manufacturers have produced such lenses (*Table 2.1*). In 1994 only those listed as manufactured by Nikon, Olympus and Polaroid are still sold, together with the Zeiss 25 mm Luminar.

Numerical apertures (NAs) matching the various maximum $f$ numbers are:

| | |
|---|---|
| $f1.9 = NA\ 0.27$ | $f2.0 = NA\ 0.24$ |
| $f2.5 = NA\ 0.20$ | $f2.8 = NA\ 0.18$ |
| $f3.2 = NA\ 0.15$ | $f3.5 = NA\ 0.14$ |
| $f4.0 = NA\ 0.12$ | $f4.5 = NA\ 0.11$ |
| $f5.6 = NA\ 0.09$ | $f6.3 = NA\ 0.08.$ |

Diameters of fields of view for a selection of lenses *in actual use* are as follows.

(a) For Zeiss lenses with a Leitz macro-dia illuminator, with matching condensers (but a 25 mm condenser for the 16 mm lens):

| | |
|---|---|
| 16 mm Luminar | 9 mm |
| 25 mm Luminar | 14 mm |
| 40 mm Luminar | 22 mm |
| 63 mm Luminar | 37 mm |
| 100 mm Luminar | 72 mm. |

**Table 2.1:** Macro lenses

| Maker and Name | Focal length | Maximum aperture | Marked stops | Magnification range | Thread |
|---|---|---|---|---|---|
| Leitz SUMMAR | 24 | $f3.2$ | 2–12 | 4–25 × | RMS |
| and MILAR* | 35 | $f3.2$ | 2–12 | 2–16 × | RMS |
| (1960s) | 42 | $f3.2$ | 2–12 | 1.7–13 × | RMS |
| | 50* | $f3.2$ | 2–12 | 1.4–12 × | RMS |
| | 65* | $f3.2$ | 2–24 | 1.1–9 × | RMS |
| | 80 | $f4.5$ | 2–24 | 0.9–7 × | M26/0.75 |
| | 100* | $f4.5$ | 2–24 | 0.8–5 × | M34/0.75 |
| | 120 | $f4.5$ | 2–96 | 0.7–4 × | M34/0.75 |
| Leitz PHOTAR | 12.5 | $f1.9$ | $f1.9$–$f8$ | 15–30 × | RMS |
| (1970s) | 25 | $f2.5$ | $f2.5$–$f16$ | 7–16 × | RMS |
| | 50 | $f4.0$ | $f4$–$f32$ | 3–8 × | RMS |
| | 50 | $f2.8$ | $f2.8$–$f22$ | 3–8 × | RMS |
| | 80 | $f4.5$ | $f4.5$–$f32$ | 1–4 × | M40/0.75 |
| | 120 | $f5.6$ | $f5.6$–$f32$ | 0.5–2 × | M40/0.75 |
| Nikon | 19 | $f2.8$ | 1–6 | 15–40 × | RMS |
| MACRO-NIKKOR | 35 | $f4.5$ | 1–6 | 8–20 × | RMS |
| | 65 | $f4.5$ | 1–6 | 3.5–10 × | M39/10 |
| | 120 | $f6.3$ | 1–7 | 0.5–4 × | M39/1.0 |
| Olympus | 20 | $f2$ | $f2$–$f16$ | 5–13 × | OM bayonet |
| ZUIKO-MACRO | 38 | $f2.8$ | $f2.8$–$f22$ | 2.5–6.5 × | OM bayonet |
| | 80 | $f4.0$ | $f4.0$–$f32$ | 1–3 × | OM bayonet |

(These lenses are true macro lenses, in spite of their auto-iris mounts (earlier versions of 20 and 38 were non-auto RMS); they can be used with adapters on any size of camera.)

| | | | | | |
|---|---|---|---|---|---|
| Polaroid MP-4 | 17 | $f4.0$ | $f4.0$–$f22$ | 10–34 × | M40/0.75 |
| | 35 | $f4.5$ | $f4.5$–$f32$ | 5–14.8 | M40/0.75 |
| | 50 | $f4.5$ | $f4.5$–$f32$ | 3.5–10 | M40/0.75 |
| | 75 | $f4.5$ | $f4.5$–$f32$ | 1.5–7 × | M40/0.75 |
| | 105 | $f4.5$ | $f4.5$–$f32$ | 1–5 × | M40/0.75 |
| | 135 | $f4.5$ | $f4.5$–$f32$ | 0.75–3 × | M40/0.75 |
| Zeiss LUMINAR | 16 | $f2.5$ | 1–30 | 10–40 × | RMS |
| | 25 | $f3.5$ | 1–30 | 6.3–25 × | RMS |
| | 40 | $f4.5$ | 1–30 | 4–16 × | RMS |
| | 63 | $f4.5$ | 1–30 | 2–10 × | RMS |
| | 100 | $f6.3$ | 1–30 | 0.8–8 × | M44/0.75 |

(b) For Nikon lenses with the Nikon macro-dia illuminator, with matching condensers:

| | |
|---|---|
| 19 mm Macro-Nikkor | 9 mm |
| 35 mm Macro-Nikkor | 24 mm |
| 65 mm Macro-Nikkor | 52 mm |
| 120 mm Macro-Nikkor | 110 mm. |

(c) For Zeiss lenses on a compound microscope, illuminated by a Nikon macro-illuminator, NA 0.32, immediately below the stage, fields of view are:

16 mm Luminar 9 mm
25 mm Luminar 23 mm
40 mm Luminar 23 mm (Field of view limited by the condenser).

The diameter of the field illuminated by the macro illuminator is 23 mm. The same lenses used similarly with a Watson macro illuminator give the same results, as the field illuminated by this condenser is also 23 mm.

Some other suitable lenses include *high-quality* enlarger lenses, and possibly some prime lenses (*not zoom types*) of normal focus in C mounts for 16 mm or 35 mm cine work. For low magnifications, the former are used as normal (i.e. right way round with the rear element facing the negative); for high magnifications (with longer lens-to-film distance than lens-to-object) they are reversed. It is a help if they can be fitted to a shutter; in this case, if stopped down, it is necessary that their own irises be used, and not that of the shutter (which would not control the aperture, but would merely vignette). Cine lenses will almost always need reversing, to keep the conjugate distances to their calculated ratios. Reversing any lens is a simple matter if it has a threaded front mount, and especially if it is known what thread form this is. A double-threaded adapter screws into this front mount, and then into the camera body or shutter (possibly via a T-mount adapter if the body has a bayonet mount) to hold the rear of the lens forwards towards the object. Some camera makers supply such adapters, often for bellows use, but if not a wide range is available elsewhere commercially (e.g. SRB Film Service, see Appendix). It is stressed that such use of unspecialized lenses should always be regarded as a second-best option, until tested under conditions of use photographically with a target such as an England finder, and the resulting negative evaluated ruthlessly.

Close-up (supplementary) lenses have some uses occasionally in macro-range work. The 80 mm Olympus lens is supplied with a matching supplementary lens for use in special circumstances, and the combination tests well. If circumstances dictate, a positive lens can be fitted in front of a camera lens to provide a greater image scale, but the increase in magnification is minimal, and this is best seen as an expediency. It is worth noting that any lens can be fixed in front of another, to act as a supplementary lens; even a large zoom lens could be used in this way. This is *not* recommended – the fewer the number of glass surfaces used in lenses for this kind of work, the better the results always are.

## 2.5 Unsuitable lenses

Unsuitable lenses for normal or reversed use include all zoom types (which are complicated in construction and easily create flare when used in non-standard applications). Some zoom lenses (especially for 35 mm cameras) are stated by their makers to have a macro capacity; this means only that they will focus closer than usual, but they are not macro lenses in any scientific (as opposed to commercial) sense.

A number of camera manufacturers also supply prime lenses which they designate as macro, usually because they focus to 1:1 (for copying and close-up work), right way round, with or without an extension tube. These are of relatively simple construction (which is a recommendation), are well suited to their stated purpose, and may well be suitable for use with bellows some way beyond a magnification of × 1, but they are not necessarily suitable for high magnifications. Only a specific test (reversed and not) will provide proper evaluation. A few prime lenses apart from this type may also perform adequately when reversed; in general, they will be of moderate aperture and normal focal length, but their use is really only an expediency.

## 2.6 Supporting the lens

### 2.6.1 Rigid tubes

Following the advice given in Sections 2.4 and 2.5 for choosing a lens for macro-range work, attention must be given to its support in suitable equipment. A basic choice is between rigid extension tubes and more flexible bellows. Where absolute rigidity is required, as in some motion-picture work with living organisms in studio aquaria, for example, the most successful arrangement is to have each required magnification achieved by the chosen lens mounted in a specially made tube of correct length, in front of the chosen camera (which may be a video unit, a 16 mm camera, a 35 mm camera, or even one using 70 mm film for IMAX). It follows that a special tube must be machined for each magnification, and while few carrying out more general work will contemplate such an outlay in time and other resources, such an arrangement cannot be bettered, when supported on the massive framing already mentioned.

For some more general purposes, extension tubes attached to a camera body remain ideal. Usually, the required magnifications are towards the lower end of the macro range, and the prime requirement is for easy and prompt manoeuvring in the field; further consideration will be given to this subject in Chapter 4. In addition to 35 mm equipment, such tubes are available for medium-format cameras, and serious work is possible with such apparatus. Good-quality extension tubes, such as the auto tubes by Nikon and other makers, will also transmit the automatic control of the diaphragm. A special extension tube is the Olympus 65-116 Auto Tube, which offers excellent continuously variable extensions between those values, with great rigidity and maintenance of diaphragm control.

### 2.6.2 Bellows

The more flexible approach is the use of bellows. In the past these were often large (perhaps taking plates 6.5 × 8.5 inches, with an extension of over 1 m), carried on a horizontal optical bench. Nowadays there is no need to have bellows longer than 500 mm, and most work is done within a length of 300 mm. Such bellows can be purpose-made (e.g. by Camera Bellows, see Appendix) or provided in the form of an existing large-format camera, or as accessories to medium-format or 35 mm cameras; the author's 35 mm units are manufactured by Nikon and by Olympus, and both are solid and lockable; the use of a twin cable release allows the auto-iris to function in each case. Additional insertable units are available to extend the overall length if necessary.

Purpose-made set-ups have much to commend them if space is available, and some machining facilities are to hand. The best arrangement is to have the bellows mounted vertically on some kind of optical bench, which may be extended downwards to carry a stage, or may be fitted over a horizontal table to support a stage and illumination train. If this is done, the table should be about 800 mm square, heavy and levelled, and low to the floor – a height of about 300 mm is ideal. This enables adjustments to be made to the stage while kneeling or sitting on a low bench, and the ground-glass to be viewed while standing. Both ends of the bellows should be adjustable to and fro, but there is rarely a need for rise/fall and lateral movements; it is better that the lens and rear standards should be truly rigid when in use, although for reflected-light work some swing movement can be very helpful in maximizing depth of field. It is easy to make suitable standards, incorporating fittings from an old camera to avoid some complicated processes. Slightly oversize bellows are always to be preferred (perhaps 150 mm square for a $4 \times 5$ inch back); this can be made to rotate or at least to be insertable in two directions, which will save much adjustment to the objects being photographed.

If an existing technical camera is to be used (the most usual solution nowadays, since none of the older bench-type special cameras is now sold), it should be supported (truly) vertically and attached to some kind of optical bench. If a Sinar monorail-type camera is used, two clamps for the rail should be used for rigidity, and if a baseboard-type camera (e.g. Linhof or Wista) is used, provision should be made to have it attached with two spaced screws rather than the usual single screw (*Figure 2.3*). A vertically mounted, triangular-section, student-type, 1 m optical bench is very suitable for this purpose, the usual saddles being very handy attachments by which to carry a camera. If a solid wall is not available to attach such a bench, suitably braced steel scaffolding tubing (as already mentioned) can be set up in the middle of a room if need be (this actually offers advantages of access, especially for lighting), providing suitable anchorages are available top and bottom. The optical bench can be attached directly to the basic support, or carried on anti-vibration mounts (with the bench below carried separately) if need be. If a baseboard camera is used in this way, it should be held proud of the optical bench on heavy steel spacers; otherwise, its optical axis might be too close to the wall or supporting framework to allow a macro-dia illuminator to be used below.

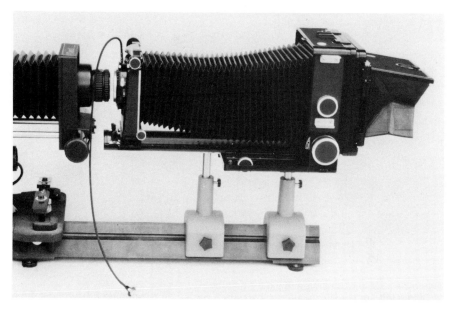

**Figure 2.3:** Adequate support for occasional macro work.

When having to use a lash-up, proper support of the camera of whatever format requires use of more than one carrier. The Wista camera shown here has two supports on an ordinary triangular-section optical bench; it has the longer bellows in place, with the longer bed also. Also attached to the bench, on an old microscope platform for such a bench, is a Durst M670 ($6 \times 7$ cm) condenser enlarger-head, which is being used evenly to light a large histological slide and to form the image with its 105 mm El-Nikkor lens. The Copal 1 shutter contains no lens, of course. This is a versatile set-up for photographing large sections, which are very difficult to light evenly otherwise. It would be equally possible to use a 100 mm macro lens in the camera shutter, if one was to hand, and none in the enlarger; the enlarger bellows would still be extended to reduce glare, and the whole is operated in a darkened room.

For purely 35 mm work, perhaps for lecture slides only, 35 mm bellows can be used. All the major manufacturers make them to suit their own equipment (Olympus in particular make a very full range of macro equipment), and general-purpose bellows are also available, generally more cheaply (*Figure 2.4*). It is always best to have high-quality bellows which have adjustable (and locking) standards at both ends, and which can be moved *in toto* on a further rail once set (for focusing, if the stage does not itself focus). There is also much to be said for having 35 mm equipment mounted on bellows intended for a larger format. If a $4 \times 5$ inch camera is the basic installation, it is easy to provide an adapter plate for the rear, perhaps fitting this instead of the usual $4 \times 5$ inch darkslide, and carrying an adapter to take the desired 35 mm camera body. The already available macro lenses are then used for 35 mm work also, and the extra solidity of the larger unit is a positive advantage. A short extension tube may be needed between the plate and the body, to allow the head to approach the

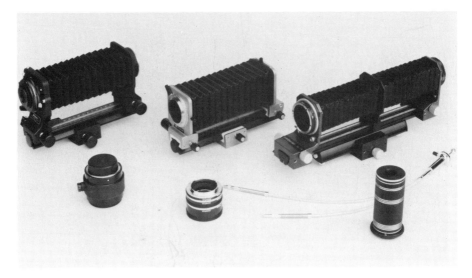

**Figure 2.4:** 35 mm bellows and extension tubes.
On the left are the Nikon auto-bellows PB-6, carried on a clamping focusing rail. Both standards of the bellows also focus and clamp (an extension bellows PB-6E is also available). The front standard is carrying an adapter for RMS-threaded macro lenses. In front is the long Nikon auto extension ring PN-11. In the middle are the Olympus auto-bellows, carried on a clamping focusing rail and with clamping standards back and front. In front of them is a set of Olympus auto extension tubes, in lengths of 7, 14 and 25 mm. On the right are the Alpa bellows, non-automatic, with the longer clamping focusing rail and extension bellows in place. Front and rear standards both clamp, and adapters are readily added to accommodate any make of lens and any make of camera body. A set of Alpa non-auto extension tubes is in front, fitted with the RMS thread adapter for macro lenses. A double cable release is shown, of the kind necessary to operate with auto-bellows to close the iris in advance of operating the shutter.

viewfinder in comfort, and all the automatic exposure functions of the body are available in the normal way (*Figure 2.5*).

## 2.7 Camera movements

Camera movements are sometimes useful in reflected-light work, but to only a very small extent for actual positioning of the image. When it is realized that moving a camera standard a distance of 5 mm moves the image on the film a distance of 5 mm, and that one may be working at a magnification of $\times 10$, it is very easy to lose sight of a specimen completely by using camera movements in macro-range photography, even if they are smooth enough to be used at all. Control of position is usually best achieved by moving the specimen stage, but for initial alignment of a system for transmitted-light work, camera movements can be useful (see Section 2.8). It has already been said that some swing is useful on both standards to

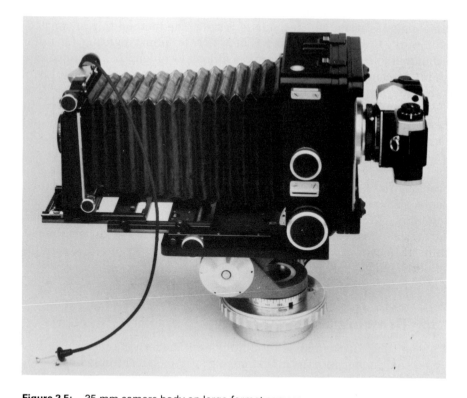

**Figure 2.5:** 35 mm camera body on large-format camera.

A Wista camera is shown, with a Copal shutter having the RMS adapter for a macro lens. At the rear, a plate carrying a thread to accept any camera-body adapter has been attached, using the clamps provided to accept a roll-film back. The plate was made up in the workshop, and is fully light-tight. In place is shown an Olympus OM4Ti body. This makes an excellent heavy-duty bellows unit for a 35 mm back; it is free from glare on account of its large size and allows any macro lens to be used, with camera movements if necessary. The shutter is provided with adapters to accept all makes of macro and enlarging lenses. As with all bellows, the use of a cable release at least 20 cm long is vital.

maximize depth of field in reflected-light work, according to the Schiempflug rule. (This requires theoretical extensions of the planes of object, lens panel and film to meet at a point if maximum depth of field is to be obtained, and is further discussed by Langford (1986).)

## 2.8 Compound systems for macro-range work

### 2.8.1 Low-power objectives

It is possible, and in some circumstances desirable, to obtain magnifications of $\times 10$ and upwards using an ordinary compound microscope with $\times 1$, $\times 2$ or $\times 4$ objectives and a $\times 10$ eyepiece. If this is done, the working distance is usually very much smaller than with a macro lens giving the same magnification, which tends to restrict the method to transmitted-light work, there being no space in which to adjust lighting for other techniques. Very few older objectives in long focal lengths give adequate quality in comparison with macro lenses, and the method is useful only with modern coated objectives. For example, the $\times$ 1/NA 0.04 and $\times$ 2/NA 0.08 S-Plan Fluorite, and $\times$ 4/NA 0.16 S-Plan Apochromatic objectives in the Olympus LB series, used with the Olympus Ultra-low Condenser and a $\times$ 2.5 NFK photo-eyepiece, give excellent results (with a relay lens to project the image into the film plane); the fields of view have diameters of 20, 11 and 6 mm respectively, thus comparing well with macro lenses of focal lengths 40 and 25 mm. Other manufacturers produce modern equivalents, such as the $\times$ 1.25/NA 0.04, $\times$ 2.5/NA 0.075 and $\times$ 5/NA 0.16 Plan-Neofluars of Zeiss, with working distances of 3.5, 9.3 and 12.2 mm, respectively. Some large modern multi-purpose stands produce automatically low-power macrographs, in both 35 mm and large formats, perhaps simultaneously.

## 2.8.2  Drawing tubes

Drawing tubes are available for a number of modern stands. Since they project their image into the main imaging system, if a suitably lit slide (or even a suitably lit solid object) is imaged with such a tube, and no image is present in the main tube, it is possible to obtain a very low-power picture (perhaps not of the highest quality) by this means, which should not be overlooked in an emergency.

## 2.8.3  Stereo microscopes

These are available nowadays in many configurations, and a camera (usually only 35 mm) can be attached to one or other eyetube of most for the cost of a simple adapter, the built-in focusing and exposure devices of the camera being used to make low-power pictures. This is a very convenient way to make occasional macrographs, but they may lack a certain quality unless the best type of instrument is chosen. This is of the common front objective type, when one tube is used to take all the image straight through (i.e. without prisms in train). If such an instrument is used, with zoom system if incorporated, then results can be good and simple to obtain.

## 2.8.4  Macroscopes

Macroscopes as such were introduced in the late 1960s, with the Zeiss Tessovar. Originally for use with a Contarex 35 mm camera, it was used

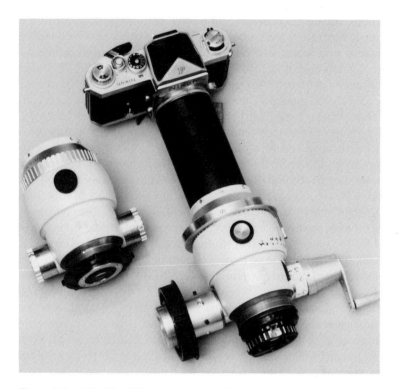

**Figure 2.6:** (Modified) Tessovar zoom units.
On the left is a relatively unmodified unit, with a different front installed. On the right of the plate, the unit's zoom control has been extended at each side – on the left with a gear for motor drive, and on the right with a long handle and new markings for more precise control at some distance. This unit carries modular extension tubes and a Nikon F Camera body, used for stills to record the kinds of pictures normally made in motion. The Tessovar zoom units are ideal for incorporating into purpose-built equipment, and a good workshop is a vital part of a good macro-range studio. A feature of the arrangements of the Image Quest 3D Ltd studio is the modular nature of the equipment, all specially made, and all easily assembled to suit specific requirements. Photograph made by kind permission of Peter Parks.

(and, by some, is still) for other formats, especially for motion pictures (*Figure 2.6*). In one setting, the iris does not vary the intensity throughout the zoom range of 4:1, a real boon when filming. It incorporates a front circle of four openings with RMS threads, housing supplementary lenses of powers $\times 0.25$, $\times 0.5$ and $\times 2$ (with one blank), to give a total range of $\times 0.4$–12.6 on 35 mm film at four working distances (between 36 and 250 mm). The numerical aperture of the system is low (and not suited to transmitted-light work with slides), but a standard low-power objective can be used in the blank position, and this can modify results dramatically. The instrument incorporates a prism viewfinder (with attachable telescope for focusing low powers), and a rather coarse helical focusing.

The Wild M400 series PhotoMakroskop was introduced in the early 1980s, specifically as an automatic piece of equipment for photography in the macro range. The original M400 had a fixed camera port, accepting a 35 mm back or a $4 \times 5$ inch back above the viewing tubes, below which a $5 : 1$ zoom system was found which could be used with three supplementary lenses ($\times 0.5$, $\times 1.5$ and $\times 2$) to give an overall range of $20 : 1$. Later versions allow users to attach their own camera bodies (M420), or are for viewing only (M410) (*Figure 2.7*). A variable beam-splitter can direct all the light to the camera tube from the single common objective, giving good-quality pictures even with transmitted illumination of histological slides. Magnifications in the film plane with 35 mm are $\times 1.3$–25.6, with field diameters from 53 mm to 2.6 mm. With a $4 \times 5$ inch back magnifications are $\times 4$–68; for direct viewing (with $\times 10$ eyepieces) they are $\times 4$–80 (but $\times 15$ and $\times 20$ eyepieces are also available). With the M400 fully automatic version comes a control box of considerable completeness, allowing control of exposure over a very wide range, allowing for minute adjustments in film speeds, for darkground work and for easy calibrating; the 35 mm back has automatic wind-on, of course. A different automatic 35 mm back and control module is available for the M420 version, and here a choice of projection eyepieces is possible as one is inserted below the shutter unit. The same choice of projection eyepiece is available for non-automatic cameras (including $4 \times 5$ inch), and it is a considerable advantage to be able to vary the magnification on the film, apart from varying the main controls. Various accessories are made for this excellent instrument, and some will be described below.

## 2.9 Comparative merits of single-lens and compound systems

The comparative merits of single-lens and compound systems revolve largely around the working distance. For example, using the three Olympus objectives mentioned above ($\times 1$, $\times 2$ and $\times 4$), the working distances are 2.2, 5.5 and 9.8 mm respectively, which are much smaller than the corresponding macro lenses for similar magnifications (the Summar 24 is about 20 mm and, the Summar 35 about 36 mm), and in inverse order of focal length into the bargain! There is little to choose in image sharpness and contrast and, for transmitted-light work with stained sections, it may be that a compound system of such quality is easier to use (and perhaps more widely or easily available than a macro system). For reflected-light work, however, where lamps must be positioned perhaps at a high angle to light a cavity, the macro system is the only choice, for there is just not enough working space to adjust such lighting using a low-power objective.

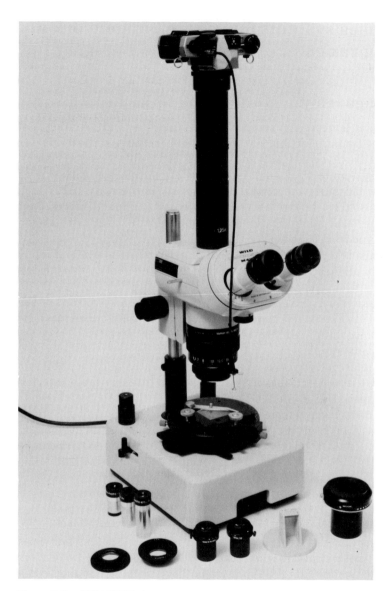

**Figure 2.7:** Wild M420 photomacroscope.

The unit is shown on the illuminating base, with built-in power supply, three condensers and ground-glass, and intensity control. This carries the polarizing stage with attached mechanical stage. The camera tube has a factor of × 1.5, and is here fitted with the Olympus OM4Ti camera body, which provides its own spot metering. The projection eyepiece (KPS × 2.5, × 3.2 and × 5) fitted in the tube makes the image on the film parfocal with that in the binocular viewing tubes, and gives some control of final image size. On 35 mm film, the range of magnifications is × 6.3 to × 32. Two bayonet-in supplementary lenses are shown in front (three are available: × 0.5, × 1.5 and × 2), to give an overall range of × 3.2 to × 64. An extra pair of eyepieces (× 20/13) is shown, interchangeable with the × 10/21 usually used. Next to these in the plate is the mirror device used to align the lamp, and next to that is the shutter for the rigid 4 × 5 inch. back; that used by the author is the one supplied with the Olympus BHS microscope. The unit can be mounted horizontally (see *Figure 4.5*), and also on a universal arm capable of placing it over a wide radius with precision and rigidity.

# 2.10 Lenses/systems for macro-range work at long range

## 2.10.1 Image relay

In some cases it is necessary to obtain quite highly magnified images at some distance from the action (e.g. if high temperatures, radioactivity or shy creatures are involved). To some extent it is possible to arrange for an image-relay system to work surprisingly well in such cases, certainly as an emergency measure where such work is rare. In the early 1920s such a system was sold by a particular London dealer who made extravagant claims for the total magnifications obtainable in this way (the Davon microscope), and from time to time the idea has been revamped. Basically, an aerial image is formed by one system, and then further magnified by another. As in all optical magnification systems, the quality depends on what the very first lens achieves, later lenses being able only to try to correct or make more convenient what was achieved at the front of the optical train. On the other hand, by careful choice of components, the working distance for a high magnification can be arranged to be surprisingly long. At its simplest, if a microscope is set up horizontally, and a good-quality telescope objective of about 150 mm focus and about 30 mm aperture is set into a suitable tube with two or three suitable internal diaphragms spaced to minimize flare, and this is held in the substage collar, it can be focused to form an aerial image in the plane of the stage. If this image is then magnified with a low-power objective and eyepiece in their usual places in the body tube, a magnification of up to $\times 50$ can be obtained, with a focusing range from about 2 m to infinity. The same results may be obtained experimentally with a monorail camera or optical bench with adequate quality, provided that flare is avoided at the first image plane by shielding the optical path. Experimenting with various (low-power) objectives gives a range of magnifications, although the images are not very bright. A thermometer scale is readable at 5 m, and gives a magnification of $\times 25$ at 2 m when using a $\times 10$ eyepiece and $\times 4$ objective; a large garden spider fills a 35 mm frame in these circumstances. If a 100 mm objective is used in a suitable substage tube, with a $\times 10$ eyepiece and $\times 4$ objective on the body tube, magnifications of about $\times 50$ are obtained at about 300 mm. It must be emphasized that the optical quality of the images is adequate but not excellent, but when necessary they give useful information when no other method can be used. It is also possible to use a modification of the system to place a close-up in front of a distant view, although this is tending towards the film-makers' special effects department (Mesner, 1990).

## 2.10.2 Questar

The Questar Maksutov-Cassegrain telescope (The Questar Corporation, see Appendix) in its smallest size (3.5 inch aperture) has long been a favourite excellent-quality compact instrument for astronomy and also for terrestrial use and high-power telephotography; 35 mm cameras can be attached very easily, and it has an effective visual focal length of about 1400 mm in this form (but 2800 mm photographically). If the camera is attached on an extension tube or two, the effective focal length is increased without noticeable diminution in quality, as its resolution is so high (*Figure 2.8*). Although its focusing range comes as close as 10 feet, it was not intended for closer range work. Nonetheless, with 16 mm cine film, the author has filled the frame with an ant at approximately 5 m. A modified version, the Questar M1, is specifically intended for work in the range 22–77 inches, with an aperture of $f14.4$. With a 35 mm camera, the field covered ranges between 10 and 58 mm, respectively, with a resolution of 128 lines mm$^{-1}$ on axis; visually, the magnification varies from $\times 22$ to $\times 8$, respectively, with a 25 mm eyepiece (others can be used). With a small video camera, the field covered lies between 4 and 13 mm. The optics pass wavelengths from 330 to 1500 μm, which is a very useful wide range for

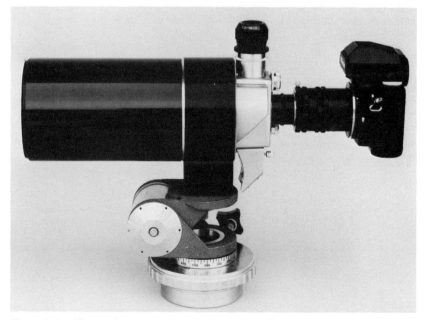

**Figure 2.8:** 'Questar' set up for close-range work.
The instrument, in field (as opposed to astronomical) mode, is supported on a Sinar pan-and-tilt head (the best design the author has used). A Nikon F3 camera body is attached to the camera port, on Questar extension tubes. In this mode, at a distance of 3.5 m, the long side of the 35 mm format included a field of 75 mm, a magnification of just less than $\times 0.5$ at this considerable working distance. Image quality is superb, and by adding further tubes or flicking in the Barlow lens greater magnification is at once secured, without noticeable diminution in apparent resolution.

photographic work. The instrument is jewel-like in build, about 300 mm long with a diameter of about 110 mm, and weighing less than 2 kg. All focusing movements are internal, and the eyepiece is on a right-angle elbow at the rear, out of the way of the attached camera on-axis; a flip of a lever moves between the two. In view of its high magnifications, it must be supported on a heavy tripod or other support, to minimize vibration effects. A camera body with shutter prerelease is recommended (or use a self-timer) for the same reason. Such an instrument is not cheap, but for situations where much long-range macro work has to be undertaken it is invaluable.

### 2.10.3 Katoptaron

The Katoptaron LDM-1 is another catadioptric macro lens, with a primary mirror 3.5 inches in diameter and a focusing range from 80 cm to infinity (H. Hakowsky, see Appendix). Although the author has not worked with an example, it is reported to be slightly less easy to handle than the Questar, with the camera attached behind and perhaps a binocular head on top. A special feature is that the mirrors adjust sideways to control spherical and other aberrations. The effective focal length is 750 mm when used at an object distance of 1500 mm. At this distance, the magnifications obtained vary from $\times 2.5$ with a $\times 5$ eyepiece, to $\times 10$ with a $\times 20$ eyepiece. An accessory increases these values to a range of $\times 12.5\text{--}50$.

# References

**Langford M.** (1986) *Basic Photography*, 5th edn. Focal Press, London, pp. 108–110.

**Mesner WL.** (1990) Aerial image relay: a multiplane focusing technique. *J. Biol. Photography* **58**, 95–101.

# 3 Working with Transmitted Light

The requirements in both equipment and technique for work in the macro range with transmitted illumination are quite different from those needed for reflected-light work, although what was said in Chapter 2 about obtaining the required magnifications – types of camera and lens – generally applies to both.

## 3.1 The choice of illumination systems

There are three main kinds of system. The first is the macro-dia illuminator base, with lamphouse and interchangeable condensers to suit the macro lenses used. The second is a range of bases supplied for stereo microscopes and/or purpose-made macroscopes. The third is a more makeshift apparatus, which is portable and used only occasionally.

## 3.2 Macro-dia illuminators

### 3.2.1 Leitz Aristophot

Macro-dia illuminator bases are available from only a few makers, but may occasionally be available second-hand. In addition to the unit itself, large and heavy stands (which can carry compound microscopes as well as macro gear) and cameras (35 mm and large-format) were offered as part of the whole set-up. As an example, the earlier (1960s) Leitz Aristophot equipment is a basic twin-pillar stand with a single focusing bar, designed to accept a 4 × 5 inch reflex camera or to carry a 35 mm Leica with a Visoflex attachment. The macro-dia apparatus is finished in black, and is noticeably smaller than later versions (*Figure 3.1*). It consists of a baseplate carrying an Ortholux lamphouse at the side, and a mirror-housing with stage (160 × 150 mm) on top; the stage focuses smoothly and positively by rack-and-pinion from a lateral prismatic bar. The stage has the very useful

**31**

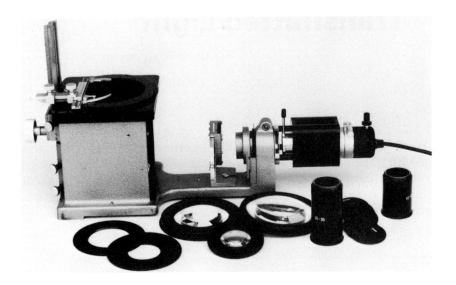

**Figure 3.1:**    The Leitz Aristophot macro-dia apparatus base (1960s model).
The smallish base has the usual Leitz lamphousing, with centring lampholder and focusing collector lens. The attachable polarizing filter holder is seen in position on the base. An attachable mechanical stage (from a Leitz microprojector) has been incorporated. In front are some of the interchangeable condensers (matching the various focal lengths of the macro lens), some of the larger and smaller apertures, and two extension tubes, intended for use with the tungsten macro-light illuminator. The lens is set at a height above the condenser in the top of the unit (below the stage) to secure magic-lantern-type illumination (with the focus inside the macro lens), and the object is focused by moving the stage by the rear knob. This is an excellent piece of apparatus, and if available second-hand should not be missed.

feature of a rotating central plate; to this (with a little ingenuity) may be attached a suitable mechanical stage, above the recess for the stage masks, a set of which provides openings varying from 15 to 80 mm diameter in nine steps, as required to match the specimen being photographed. Below this level an interchangeable condenser (matching the lens in use, and marked 24, 35, 42, 65, 80, 100 or 120) is fitted. A mirror at 45° reflects the illumination, which comes from the 6V 30W tungsten lamp in a centring holder with a focusing collector. A swing-in supplementary lens is used with longer focal lengths, and a slide-in polarizer can be attached on its own carrier (the analyser is carried in a collar over the macro lens, via matching adapter rings). An iris may be added in front of the collector lens; this is an important modification, providing proper control of the aperture in setting up (*Figure 3.2*).

A rare accessory to this apparatus is a drawing mirror, which allows images at scales from × 5 to × 25 to be projected on to a sheet of paper at bench level with the various lenses. A well made mahogany case houses all the lenses, condensers and masks very conveniently. This excellent

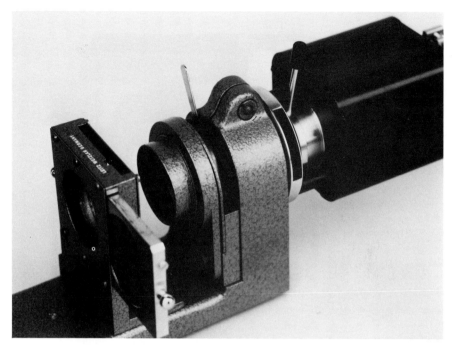

**Figure 3.2:** Insertion of an iris diaphragm in the Leitz macro-dia base.
  The focusing rod for the collector is seen on the right, behind the filter slot. A swing-out lens is fitted for use with the lenses with the longest focus, and between its housing and the clamp for the lamphouse the author has fitted an iris diaphragm to act as a field diaphragm (not included by Leitz). This is most helpful in controlling glare, and should be present in all macro illumination systems.

Aristophot macro-dia apparatus was superseded in the later 1970s by a larger version, finished in light colour, with similar accessories; this has also now been withdrawn.

## 3.2.2 Other macro-dia apparatus

The Olympus macro-dia apparatus, well made on similar lines, and intended for 35 mm use, is rather smaller, and does not have a massive stand with it. Possibly the only such unit currently available is the Multiphot by Nikon, specifically designed as a stand/diascopic base unit. The very solid stand has an antivibration rubber mat, levelling feet, twin pillars carrying a central focusing bar with front and rear standards, and bellows. These are 600 mm long for the $4 \times 5$ inch back, and either 600 or 300 mm for the 35 mm system. The front standard carries a self-cocking shutter in antivibration mount that is synchronized and speeded $1/125$ to 1 sec, and B. The rear standard carries a reflex viewing unit, and has an international $4 \times 5$ inch back, taking the usual range of darkslides and roll-film carriers, as well as Polaroid holders. The arrangement of the macro-dia base is similar to that of the Leitz unit already described, but the whole Nikon unit is much larger, finished in hammer grey, and with a stage size

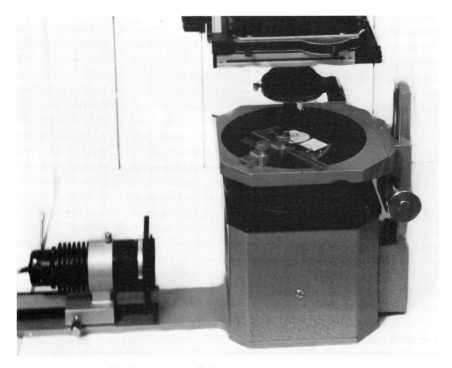

**Figure 3.3:** Nikon Multiphot macro-dia base.
The Nikon macro-dia base is still available; it is rather larger than the Leitz model but follows the same principles of providing magic-lantern-type illumination. The lamphousing moves to and fro on a dovetail, and the mirror tilts slightly, controlled by a knob, on the far side in the plate. Condensers match the four macro lenses, and the author has attached an old Leitz mechanical stage to one of the diaphragm plates. The apparatus is completely adequate (for the two middle lenses) when properly set up.

$210 \times 195$ mm (*Figure 3.3*). There is a built-in large iris in the stage, giving openings of diameters between 15 mm and 135 mm. The lamphouse slides and clamps along a dovetail, and has a 6V 30W lamp carried in a centring holder, with a focusing collector incorporating a frosted surface (not always helpful). Four multi-coated macro lenses are supplied, in focal lengths 19, 35, 65 and 120 mm. The two shorter focal lengths have RMS threads and adapters to convert to the threads (M39/1.0) of the larger; to mount on the front standard, a bayonet adapter is needed. A very important advantage of this apparatus is its mirror mounting, which has a control knob at the side that allows the mirror to be tilted. This actually provides a degree of oblique and even of darkground illumination, both techniques offering greatly increased contrast with some specimens. The author has fitted his own Multiphot lamphouse with an iris diaphragm carried on a movable plate; this allows the iris to be moved laterally in a controlled and repeatable manner to provide controlled oblique illumination (*Figure 3.4*). Four matching condensers are supplied, fitting above a condenser always in place below the stage. For the stage itself, eight aperture inserts are

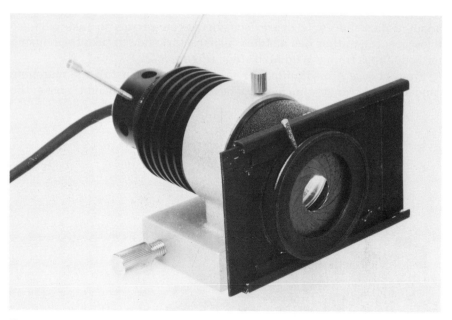

**Figure 3.4:** Multiphot lamphouse with decentrable iris diaphragm.
The author has removed the ground-glass screen from the collector-lens system of his Multiphot lamphouse, and has added a decentrable iris diaphragm, as shown. A brass plate, with grooves top and bottom, carries a further sprung plate with the wide-diameter iris attached. This can then be decentred to provide controllable and repeatable slightly oblique transmitted illumination to increase the contrast of certain objects – a valuable addition to any such system.

supplied, and the whole focuses very smoothly by rack and pinion on a rear prismatic bar. A rather crude case is offered to take the lenses and other parts, but the apparatus works very well, although the current price is breathtaking. It should not be forgotten that transmitted illumination with flash as the source may be required for living organisms; some unit having a modelling light is indispensable for accurate alignment of the system, and an image-splitter cube may be introduced to combine a tungsten source for observing the critical moment for exposure with the flash to record it to freeze the action.

# 3.3 Rigorous alignment and its importance

With all these macro-dia bases, setting up is of the greatest consequence. It is necessary that all parts of the system be accurately aligned if uneven illumination is to be avoided. Lack of evenness in illumination is observed by looking at the screen at such a distance that its whole area can be seen at once, and turning down the lamp intensity to a low level; it is very much less apparent at high lighting levels. The best method of aligning is to adapt a darkslide or a spare focusing-screen carrier to take a phase telescope; the author has adapted a spare darkslide to take the housing for body tubes from a Wild M20 stand (*Figure 3.5*).

First, choose a medium-power macro lens, and install the matching condenser. Arrange the lens to be at the correct height above the

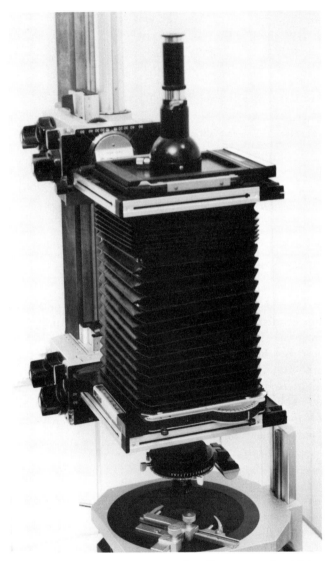

**Figure 3.5:** A phase telescope used to align a transmitted-light macro system.
The author has modified a double darkslide to take a Wild straight draw-tube. Care was taken to set the adapter accurately in the centre of the field initially, and a phase telescope is now used to view each component of the macro system in turn, to allow each to be adjusted to the optical axis. This is a prerequisite to securing even illumination of the field, at any or all focal lengths of a macro lens.

condenser, where the light cone is focused just inside the lens at the iris level (all macro-dia systems are arranged for this kind of lighting, as in a magic lantern or slide projector). Most commercial systems have their stands marked with the various heights for the several lenses, but these should always be verified as suggested above, and if a macro-dia base is being used without the same maker's camera, it will have to be done this way. Focus sharply a medium-diameter insert on the stage, and move the whole base until this is absolutely central on the screen. Install the phase telescope, and focus on the collector lens; move the mirror and/or the entire lamp until this is central. Refocus the phase telescope to the lamp filament, and centre that. Now check for evenness of lighting as suggested above. If it is uneven, adjust the distance of the lamp from the mirror, and/or adjust the focus of the lamp collector. After securing even illumination, re-check that the system is centred with the phase telescope. This procedure is carried out for every different combination of condenser and macro lens, every time a change is made, and it is thus economical when working to make photographs of all specimens requiring a particular macro lens before changing to others. The ability to focus on each level of the system in setting up is of the utmost value in securing even illumination. (The author has removed from his own Nikon lamphouse the ground-glass disc in the collector system.)

## 3.4 Recommended apparatus

### 3.4.1 Fields of view up to 20 mm diameter

In the author's experience, macro-dia equipment performs best at medium magnifications. For objects requiring fields of view up to about 20 mm diameter, the appropriate macro lens should be used with a widefield condenser and a compound microscope. This is because the illumination is excellent in such a case, the stability and freedom from vibration are better, the fine focusing required for macro lenses of short focal length is much more positive with a compound stand, and the mechanical stage allows precise positioning. The author has adapted a Wild M20 stand to take a macro lens on a special single-place nosepiece (which interchanges easily on this stand) (*Figure 3.6*). Using a standard bellows above, no cut-off is evident even at very short extensions, although a very wide diameter Sinar Copal shutter can be adapted to approach very closely by means of a light-tight trap made from wide diameter cans. For example, the three shortest focal length Zeiss Luminars and the two shortest Macro-Nikkors work very well in this way, and are usually used at one stop below maximum for transmitted-light work.

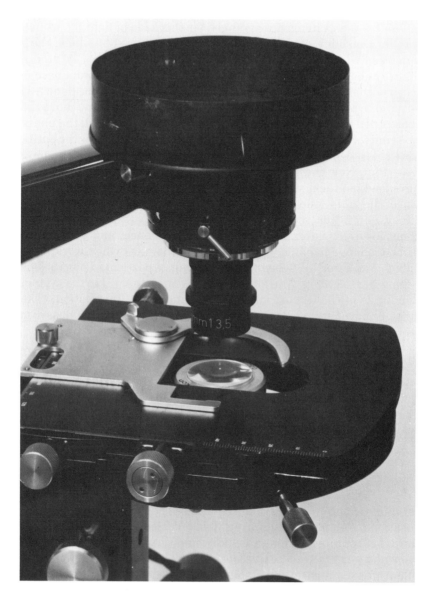

**Figure 3.6:** Compound microscope modified for use with shorter focal length macro lenses.

The author uses a Wild M20 stand for focal lengths accepting an image field of diameter up to 23 mm. An old Nikon macro illuminator is used, sitting on top of the substage ring (which it fits adequately) at stage level. The nosepiece is removed, and in its place an adapter for a single lens is fitted. Immediately above the limb, on this stand, a light-sleeve can be fitted; that made up by the author from two tin cans is very wide in diameter to match the opening in the Sinar Copal shutter and to avoid all possibility of cutting off the image. Without further effort, such a system provides built-in illumination of high intensity, filter carriers, mechanical stage, and coarse–fine focusing of great precision. This is the system which the author recommends for all such lenses of shorter focal length used with transmitted illumination.

## 3.4.2 Fields of view between 20 and 55 mm

For objects requiring a field of view of between 20 mm and 55 mm, use of the standard macro-dia equipment as above is recommended, set up carefully as described.

## 3.4.3 Fields of view greater than 55 mm

For objects requiring a field of view much in excess of 55 mm diameter, macro-dia bases can be difficult to adjust to secure even illumination. Lack of evenness may not be apparent until a final print is inspected, and it is strongly recommended that a picture is made with the lowest powers of a macro-dia apparatus carefully set up as described, but without having a specimen on the stage. Lack of even illumination is then apparent at once. If it proves impossible to secure even lighting with such equipment, recourse must be had to a different illumination system, and a $4 \times 5$ inch or a $6 \times 7$ cm condenser enlarger head (according to the size of the section) is strongly recommended. It will be described below how such an enlarger alone may be used to make macrographs. If it is more convenient to use the camera (as opposed to the enlarger alone) to make the pictures, it is not difficult to arrange the head upside down vertically, and to support the camera above in the usual way (*Figure 3.7*). Care must be taken to ensure that the ventilation slots in the head are not obstructed, and that internal components work efficiently in the inverted position. The negative carrier is used to hold the slide, which should be masked in some way to minimize glare. The enlarger lens is removed, and the bellows racked out a little way, so that the macro lens can look into them without vignetting. The author uses both sizes of enlarger head in this way, with no difficulty, by arranging that of the Durst L138 (half-plate) enlarger or of the Durst M670 (35 mm to $6 \times 7$ cm) on the levelled low bench used for supporting macro or micro equipment normally. Both are opal-lamp/condenser enlargers, with interchangeable condensers to match the lens in use. It is desirable to use a condenser that will focus the light into the macro lens used for taking the photograph, as already described for setting up a macro-dia apparatus; the phase telescope can be used for aligning, especially to make sure that the enlarger head negative carrier is truly vertical under the camera. If a longer focus macro lens is not to hand, then the (high-quality) enlarging lens itself can be used to project the image up into the camera, with the cover glass towards the lens, of course. To avoid vignetting, the lens should be placed close to the camera shutter. Either system works very well indeed, as the enlarger head was built specifically to provide even illumination of whatever size of negative it carries, and very few slides to be photographed will have a larger section on them than one measuring $4 \times 5$ inch or half-plate, and few will be larger than $6 \times 7$ cm!

As long as the distance from the slide to the lens is less than the distance from the lens to the film, the enlarger lens is inserted normally (if that is being used rather than a macro lens). If an especially large section is

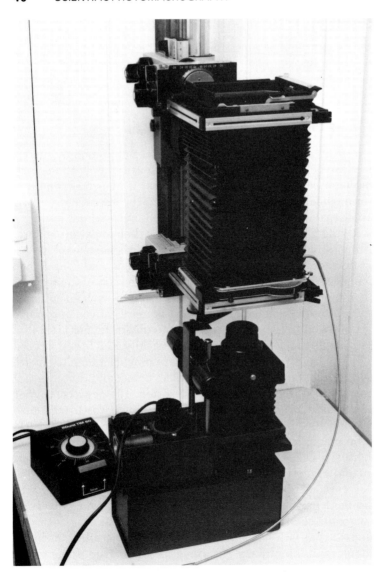

**Figure 3.7:**   Enlarger head used to form the low-power image.
The Durst M670 enlarger head readily detaches from its column in the darkroom, and stands upside down on the macro bench, below the wall-mounted Sinar camera. It is centred to the axis of the camera merely by sliding the enlarger to and fro; the 105 mm El-Nikkor high-quality enlarging lens (stopped down one stop only) forms the image, which is projected up through the Sinar Copal shutter. Alternatively, a macro lens could be used on the camera, the enlarger then providing only the even illumination for a histological or other specimen up to 6 × 7 cm in size. This system is unsurpassed for even illumination of large slides; a larger head will, of course, illuminate a larger slide.

actually being reduced at the film plane (perhaps a whole-brain section recorded on 35 mm film: a not unusual requirement that often falls to the photomacrographer), the enlarger lens must be reversed. The author uses Nikon El-Nikkor enlarging lenses, and Nikon supply little-known reversing adapters (JNW00101 for focal lengths 40–105 mm, and JNW00401 for focal lengths 135 and 150 mm) for just such a purpose, although they can be made up easily enough or obtained from specialist suppliers for other makes (e.g. SRB Film Service, see Appendix).

It is always worthwhile actually testing longer focus macro lenses also to see if they need reversing, particularly in possibly marginal conditions of image and object distances.

## 3.5 Contact printing of large preparations

Contact printing for recording very large histological slides (e.g. those of a section of an entire brain or embryo) should not be overlooked as a possibility. An enlarger is a convenient light source, with the head as high on the column as possible. If colour correction is required, this is easily performed using a colour head. If a shutter can be fitted to the lens, this will allow the quite short but normal exposure times to be controlled accurately; otherwise, a neutral-density filter may be needed below the lens to allow for sufficiently accurate timing over a few seconds. There is nothing in the negative carrier, of course, but its edges are accurately focused on to the baseboard. A sheet of film is simply placed face up on a piece of matt black velvet on the enlarger baseboard (to obviate reflection back through the film from the usually white board), the large slide is placed, cover-glass down, on top of it, and the exposure made in total darkness. The weight of the large slide usually holds the film flat but, if not, the whole is covered with a large sheet of (ultra-clean) glass. Some preliminary estimation of exposure can be made with a Sinarsix meter (see Section 3.6) used upside down, or by taking readings from a white card with a spot meter (this also checks for evenness of illumination), or by a darkroom exposure meter intended for copying. Once calibrated, this last method is the simplest of all for making photographs of large slides of excellent quality. Needless to say, the exposure time should not be lengthened for convenience by running the lamp at reduced voltage, and care should be taken not to extend the exposure for a particular film so much that it enters the reciprocity failure timings. One extra advantage of this method is that some limited 'dodging' (as in ordinary photographic printing) is possible with a difficult slide.

## 3.6 Using an enlarger to make macrographs

Using an enlarger to make photomacrographs of large slides is an excellent way to proceed, if the enlarger and its lens are of high quality. In spite of the availability of specialized macro-dia equipment from several makers, it remains difficult to obtain totally even lighting for the longer focal lengths. The use of an enlarger, a widely available apparatus specifically designed for evenly lighting a flat original, and projecting a high-quality image of it, is an obvious alternative. The slide is put into the negative carrier coverglass down, and its image projected to the baseboard as usual. If built-in masking strips are available in the carrier, they should be used; if not, it is worthwhile cutting out a mask specially to prevent light spilling round the specimen, because it will degrade the image quality if it reflects about the baseboard and walls. If sheet film is being used to record the image, it should be loaded into the usual darkslide, which is held level in position by stops (perhaps on a small board). A darkslide containing a sheet of white card is used to focus the enlarger and compose the picture. The enlarger lens should be stopped down one stop from the fully open position – any further will reduce the definition. If the lens can be fitted into a shutter, this will allow short exposures to be given with accuracy; if not, a clean neutral density filter can be put on top of the slide in the negative carrier to allow exposures of a couple of seconds to be given with sufficient accuracy. An inverted Sinarsix meter can be used to measure the background intensity as usual, or a spot meter can take readings of the background by reflection from the setting-up card. The exposure is made, of course, in total darkness. Once either method has been calibrated, total accuracy is the rule. If smaller formats are to be used, a camera body (no lens) is arranged to hold the film; it must be carried rigidly above the baseboard (probably the use of a heavy right-angle bracket of the kind used in machine-shops is best) to allow the head to be positioned so that the viewfinder can be used. Careful focusing in the viewfinder is carried out in subdued lighting, and the automatic exposure device of the camera body controls the exposure. This is always best set up to measure only the background intensity, as will be explained below; a spot meter type of camera does well for this.

## 3.7 Illuminating bases and their uses

A number of illuminating bases are available for use with either true macroscopes or with stereomicroscopes. They are often recommended by their manufacturers for transmitted-light work, and when used only visually they may be quite satisfactory. For example, the Wild M400 series of macroscopes may come with their Transmitted-light Stand EB, which is well made, with a transformer for the 6V 20W tungsten–halogen lamp and other controls in the base. The lamp is in a centring holder, and a special device is supplied for initial alignment. Three separate collector lenses of varying power may be swung-in at will by one lever. For magnifications below × 10 a swing-in frosted filter is also used to secure even illumination. Filters measuring 50 × 50 mm may be housed in a recess below the stage, and a range of easily attached stages allows for most contingencies. A gliding stage provides very smooth controllable movement even at high magnifications, and a mechanical stage is also available. One especially interesting stage is a centring rotating mechanical stage fitted for polarizing, with a rotating sensitive tint plate in a push–pull mount. When used for photomacrography, the illumination without the frosted filter is not even below about × 12 (as the manufacturer states), but the introduction of the filter definitely introduces glare and spoils the definition; this is entirely characteristic of all systems using a frosted surface in the system. Above that magnification, without the filter, the illumination is perfectly adequate, if not as good as can be obtained by other means.

A different Wild base deserves mention, since it provides darkground illumination as well as brightfield. The gliding stage also fits this base, as does a mechanical stage. A changeover lever allows direct illumination (but by a frosted glass), or puts in place a central stop, to make the tungsten–halogen illumination reflect from a peripheral segmented mirror, which provides convincing darkground illumination over a diameter of 30 mm. This is a most useful option, greatly increasing the contrast of macro images of transparent specimens (*Figure 3.8*).

## 3.8  Darkground illumination for large specimens

Darkground illumination is not difficult to obtain for large specimens up to, for example, a diameter of 150 mm although commercially available apparatus is not suitable for this procedure. The author has constructed equipment for this pupose (with thanks to D.J. Thomson for discussions), using as the main support a black plastic wastepaper bin. Holes were cut into this (with a tank cutter) low down to provide ventilation for the 12V 100W tungsten–halogen lamp, which was held in the usual simple base, supported on a platform attached to an old telescoping bullseye stand on a loaded base. A pair of wires (old bicycle spokes have the correct rigidity) were crossed above the lamp, with a central pin to take darkground discs of various sizes (up to about 150 mm). These must be covered with matt black velvet on top to make a truly black background. The base was placed inside the wastepaper bin, its weight keeping it in place, and the level of the lamp was adjusted as required to give suitable illumination. The light was reflected on to the specimen by a band of aluminium cooking foil pasted inside the top quarter of the wastepaper bin; this is easily renewable when necessary. To support the large slides normally lit in this way,

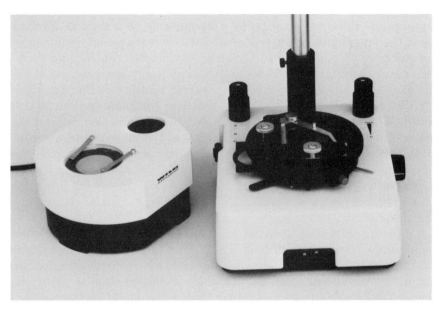

**Figure 3.8:** Wild illumination bases for transmitted-light work.
The base on the left, intended for a stereomicroscope, provides both lightfield and darkground illumination at the touch of a lever. For direct illumination, a frosted glass is automatically inserted, and for darkground a field of 30 mm diameter is well lit. Its column has been removed to allow it to be positioned below a camera. The base on the right is the transmitted-light stand EB for the Wild macroscopes; it is fitted here with the very comprehensive attachable polarizing stage, with rotating push-in, sensitive-tint plate and attached mechanical stage. The base provides illumination, via interchangeable built-in condensers, suited to the whole range of the macroscope (field diameters of 2.6–53 mm). Lower magnifications require the use of the built-in frosted glass to approach even illumination, but some glare is introduced by its use. The intensity is controlled via a knob, the lampholder centres, and there are sockets to allow reflected-light lamps to be attached to the black bases visible at the rear of the base of the instrument.

two pieces of brass channel (about 3 mm deep) were simply placed across the top of the bin (thus obviating spurious refractions from dirt on the glass plate which might otherwise have been used to support the slide). The apparatus is entirely satisfactory, and can be made up to whatever size is required (*Figure 3.9*).

An adequate darkground illumination can be provided by the macro ring illuminator from an old (black) Leitz Artistophot apparatus. This is intended for the shadowless illumination of solid objects by reflected light, but it (or a variant) works very well for darkground transmitted light. The equipment consists of a housing containing a circle of miniature low-voltage tungsten lamps; an opal screen lies under them, and two movable sectors clip in place at will (to give some directionality to the light if need be). If this equipment is used upside down, without the opal screen, with a slide or other object supported at the proper height above it, surrounded by a matt black mask laid across the top edge of the housing, the low angle of the lamps relative to a small specimen (up to about 40 mm

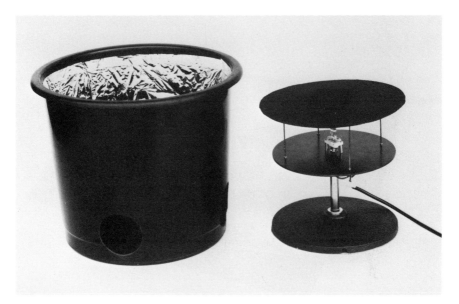

**Figure 3.9:**   Large darkground base.
A 15 l black plastic wastebin was modified to make an illuminator which will provide darkground for specimens larger than $4 \times 5$ inch without difficulty. Ventilating holes were cut into the plastic, and a band of aluminium cooking foil was glued around the top quarter of the bin. An old telescoping bullseye stand was used to take a disc of matt black Formica (an excellent constructional material), to which were attached two bent bicycle spokes and a lampbase for a 12V 100W tungsten–halogen lamp. On top, at the crossing of the wires, a pin stands to take discs of various diameters, to suit the focal length of the lens in use on the camera above. A piece of matt black velvet is used to cover the pin and, by trial and error, the correct height of the lamp is set. For this, and in use, the housing is lowered into the bin, where it is centred, by eye, on the bottom, and where it stays without movement (its base is loaded). Slides and other specimens are supported across the top of the bin by thin brass channels to avoid introducing any unwanted extra refractions from any other surfaces.

diameter) ensure that no direct light is transmitted to the macro objective (*Figure 3.10*).

Another way of securing a quasi-darkground transmitted illumination is simply to support a suitably sized (up to about 30 mm diameter) specimen at the proper height above the ringlight head of a fibre-optic illuminator. This may have a circle of outlets, or perhaps four separated outlets for the illumination, but a very satisfactory effect is obtained with great ease (*Figure 3.11*). Specially mounted ring illuminators with smaller diameters that fit at the correct height in a microscope substage are available commercially and will give good darkground to a diameter of 25 mm, with the added advantage of easy focusing and positioning. The Fostec darkfield illuminator P/N 8640 has adapters to fit Olympus BH2, Nikon Labphot and Zeiss Axioskop substages, and will illuminate a darkground field of diameter up to 25 mm at a working distance between between 0 and 10 mm.

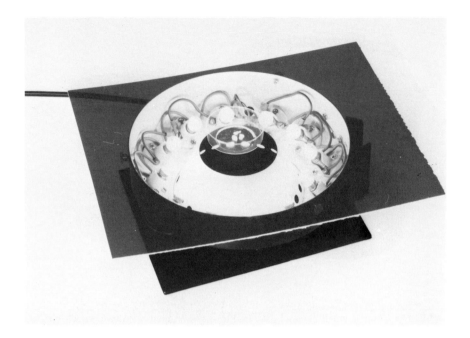

**Figure 3.10:** Inverted Leitz ring illuminator for darkground work.
  This picture was made using a split exposure. The Leitz Aristophot tungsten ring light was turned upside down, on a matt black velvet base, and covered with a sheet of black card, which supported the dish containing the crystals to be photographed. An excellent darkground effect was obtained, as all the light was reaching the subject from an acute angle. The total exposure was 10 sec; for six of these, the top card was kept in place. The 12 6V 6W krypton bulbs, wired in parallel, have been substituted for the 12 8V lamps originally wired in series. In normal use, right-way-up, a slot-on carrier holds a ground-glass diffuser, which can carry two movable sectors to give some direction to the diffuse illumination provided.

Yet another method also uses a fibre-optic illuminator. If the slide is supported relatively high, and the light from one or more (focused) light guides is directed from a shallow angle from below, only the refracted light will enter the macro lens. A matt black sheet must be placed a few centimetres below the specimen to absorb stray light. This method is also easy to arrange, works for specimens up to about 50 mm in diameter, and has the considerable additional advantage that colour filters can be introduced into one or more of the lightguides to give almost Rheinberg illumination (coloured object on a differently coloured background) on a large scale (*Figure 3.12*).

A device which has been used occasionally by the author is a slide where the balsam-mounted specimen acts as its own lightguide. Aluminium cooking foil is moulded around the lens of a fibre-optic guide at one side, and around the end of a slide at the other. The light is then carried by the slide, object, medium or cover, and the cleared object is seen very clearly

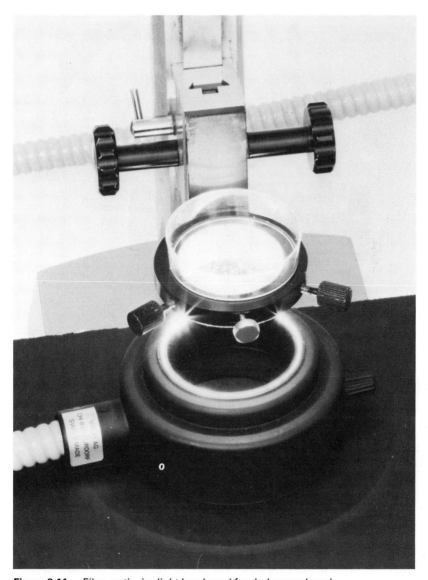

**Figure 3.11:** Fibre-optic ringlight head used for darkground work.
The ringlight head provides a continuous circle of light, intended for shadowless illumination from above; it has a definite focus. When used inverted, it is laid on a matt black background with the subject supported at a suitable distance above it to give effective darkground illumination. In the picture the subject is supported on an old inverted Prior microscope stand, and no camera is included to avoid hiding the details to be demonstrated; in practice, an aperture in a card, held at the correct height above the light, would be used to prevent glare. The ringlight shown has a wide-diameter lightguide to maximize use of the total illumination output of the source.

from above in apparent darkground mode. A very well-made, and expensive, commercial model of such an illuminator has very recently become available (Micro Video Instruments Inc., see Appendix).

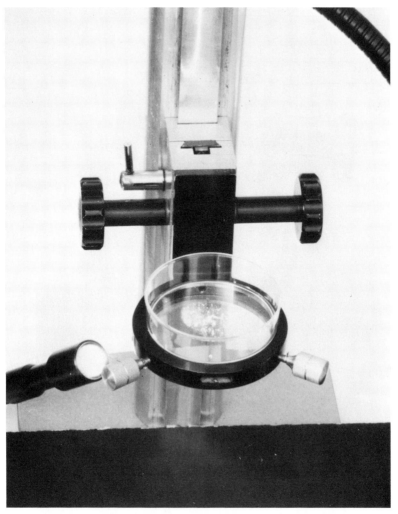

**Figure 3.12:** Fibre-optic guide to provide quasi-darkground illumination.
The same inverted Prior stand was used as in *Figure 3.11* to support the subject above a focused fibre-optic lightguide; a black card forms the background. This illumination is not true darkground, which should have a full circle of light, but it serves very well for some subjects. More than one guide can be used, of course, and each can be adjusted to give the required effect, independently of the others if need be, so the method is very flexible.

# 3.9 Temporary and portable apparatus

Occasionally, working in a well-equipped macro studio is unfeasible. Perhaps macro work is rarely undertaken, or must be undertaken away from base. In such cases suitable temporary and/or portable apparatus may be necessary. The first requirement is solid, rigid support; the

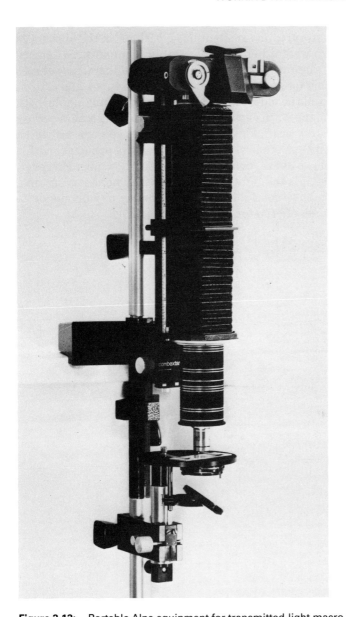

**Figure 3.13:**   Portable Alpa equipment for transmitted-light macro work.
   The Alpa 'Macrostat' equipment clamps to a bench edge, and accepts columns above and below. The bellows unit and camera body, with extra extension tubes for greater extension distance, are attached to the top side. A unit with a focusing stage and mirror and a built-in, low-power condenser is attached to the bottom. It is not suggested that such equipment should serve as a permanent set-up, but it is highly portable, light in weight, rigid in assembly and satisfactory in use.

second is accurate alignment. Some builders' scaffolding might serve as the backbone of a system, with parts clamped to this as required. A triangular-section, student-type, 1 m optical bench (often available, with its saddles, in a laboratory) is an excellent base, perhaps in the horizontal position where its own weight helps keep it stable. Standard rods attach equipment and allow alignment. Some proprietary equipment also serves if it is already available for general photography. Foba tubes and clamps are strong and rigid, and the older Alpa Macrostat can be invaluable; both offer easy camera and apparatus attachment via standard camera screws (*Figure 3.13*). Laboratory scaffolding of the Climpex type can provide a stable support. If need be, a stage clamped to a strong bench edge, with a mirror below and bellows above, can prove surprisingly stable. However, in such circumstances, it is the light source which may not be as suitable as desired; few lamps have good collectors, and it may pay dividends to check carefully any lamp offered for temporary use.

# 4 Working with Reflected Light

The image is formed using lens and camera systems as already described in Chapter 2, but for reflected-light work the support of the specimen and the way it is illuminated are very different from the requirements for transmitted-light work. It is equally necessary to maintain rigidity, but it may also be necessary to adjust the angle of viewing of the specimen by a smaller or larger amount; the small depth of field provides acute problems, and confusing shadows are easily generated. For scientific work, it is usually desirable to keep the background simple and fairly neutral in colour. Distracting shadows are almost always best avoided, often by suspending the subject high above the background so that the shadows fall outside the field of view, or by resting the subject on clean glass, plain or opal. This advice applies to all succeeding parts of this chapter.

## 4.1 Supporting tiny specimens

There is much to be said for using a compound microscope to work with the smallest specimens, as was recommended for transmitted-light work and for the same reasons: better positioning with the built-in mechanical stage; better control of focusing; and assured rigidity and alignment. Some old-fashioned accessories can be of immense use in this work. For example, the substage condenser–carrier can occasionally be used to support a dark-well of the Victorian kind; this is a very convenient holder for tiny specimens, although it means that the mechanical stage cannot be used. Alternatively, a suitable specimen holder can be used on the stage itself; a range of second-hand stage forceps and insect stages should be accumulated, or made up in the workshop over time if varied specimens are expected. Old-fashioned draughtsmens' ruling pens (of the type with screw-operated separable blades) make good stage forceps that need little adaptation. Vacuum forceps are also useful to support such tiny specimens. If a series of similar specimens is usually dealt with, special permanent holders can be devised. In the past, great ingenuity was exhibited in evolving means of specimen support when a microscopist was prepared to deal with all subjects, solid and transparent, using objectives

**51**

of focal length between 4 and $1/12$ inch. The contemporary uses of such ingenious devices can be learnt from a look through old manufacturers' catalogues and old textbooks of microscopy (Beck, 1865 (reprinted in facsimile, 1987); Carpenter, 1901).

It is usually a good idea to use a speck of Blu-tack™ or the like to make such specimens stay in place once positioned; most of the time taken in high-power, macro-range, reflected-light work is spent in adjusting the specimens properly, which move very easily indeed in face of a stray breath or accidental jarring.

The considered recommendation for the highest power reflected-light work (with lenses of focal length between 16 mm and, say, 24 mm) is to use a suitable compound microscope to support specimen and lens. Methods of illumination are discussed below in Sections 4.8, 4.9 and 4.10 and in Chapter 5, but the longest possible focal length to secure the required magnification will allow longer working distance, and thus the greatest flexibility in positioning the lamps.

## 4.2 Supporting small specimens

For mid-range macro specimens (those needing focal lengths of between about 35 mm and 65 mm, say), the recommended support is a mechanical stage on a heavy levelling base, placed below a vertical camera. Ideally, vertical movement should also be available, even if this is more difficult to arrange. For permanent set-ups having much use, motor-driven movement in three axes will save a great deal of time and effort, especially if living specimens are being pictured (Section 4.6). It is not necessary to invest a great deal of money to secure such an arrangement, as a surprising number of mechanical stages are available second-hand, taken off discarded compound microscopes if need be; they are cheap and easily altered in an average workshop. Any very heavy steel or iron plate is easily fitted with three screws as levelling feet, and the two are easily joined to make a very rigid and controllable unit for reflected-light work (*Figure 4.1*).

Supporting the specimen above stage level is usually a good idea, as it allows the lighting to be adjusted to best effect much more easily, and minimizes distracting shadows, as has been emphasized already. A range of supports can be brought to bear for these medium-sized specimens (easily made, ingenious supports are described in Croy, 1961). If available, older stage forceps of various patterns might be as useful for such specimens, as they were for even smaller ones. In addition, small crocodile clips, bent paper-clips, simple pieces of wire bent to shape, blobs of Blu-tack™, and other supports are easily made up to suit particular specimens as required. A small tilting stage is a great asset on occasion, and can be made

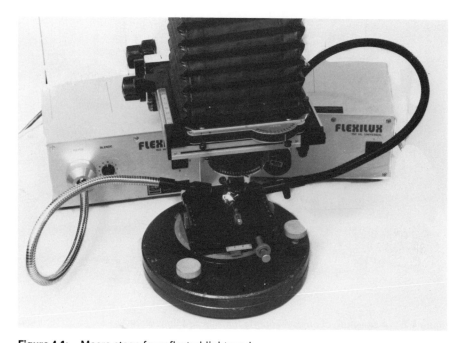

**Figure 4.1:** Macro stage for reflected-light work.
The mechanical stage from an old Russian metallurgical microscope has been attached to an old, very heavy, steel, floor-standing, levelling camera support (intended originally to facilitate making ground-level exposures with a heavy camera). This stage was stripped completely to remove the hardened lubricants, but when reassembled with modern lubricants it has proved to be a smooth and accurate support for reflected-light work, with vernier scales to both axes and to the rotation. It is shown with two fibre-optic units in use, illuminating a tiny crystal carried on an old Flatters & Garnett insect stage, to provide tilt and rotation without moving the subject out of the optical axis.

up by filling half a ping-pong (or smaller) ball with plaster (preferably mixed with carbon to minimize reflections), and supported on a rubber ring. Success in this type of photography comes from the most careful arrangement of the specimen relative to the lens and to the lighting, and more time and ingenuity than one could initially imagine will have to be expended on securing this optimum positioning. A number of insect stages have been offered in the past, and no opportunity to acquire one second-hand should ever be missed, as they allow a specimen to be positioned with some precision, especially as the stages themselves are sized to be moved bodily by a mechanical stage for precise positioning (*Figure 4.2*). If available, micromanipulator bases can provide very accurately adjustable supports for small and tiny specimens, especially if these can be attached to a fine point; easy positioning in three planes can be achieved quickly and securely by their use. Some bases (e.g. those manufactured by Prior Scientific Instruments Ltd, see Appendix) can be modified to attach to mechanical stages, to drive smaller stages in the $z$ axis, with coarse and fine focusing adaptable to motor drive; this is a very useful possibility.

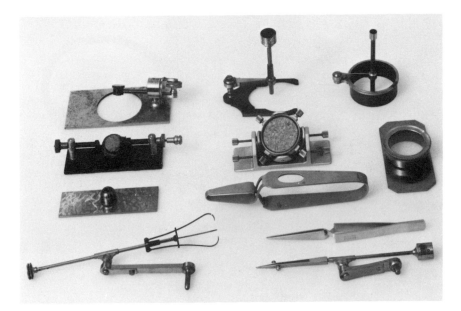

**Figure 4.2:** A selection of object supports for reflected-light work.

On the left at the back is an old (1860s) Beck opaque disc revolver. This accepts stemmed discs (diameter of 3 or 4 mm) that carry the specimens into a socket on a horizontal arm. The disc revolves via a fusee chain and knob, and also tilts; the carrier allows a Lieberkühn to be used. Such a device is not common, but should never be missed if seen second hand. In front is a Flatters & Garnett insect stage, with a cork disc which tilts and rotates in the optical axis. In front of that is an old (1880s) ball-and-socket stage, with a hole to take a pin to carry the specimen, allowing tilting in all directions. At the rear are two dark-well holders, one to fit a substage; the dark-wells accept tiny objects and allow a Lieberkühn to be used. In front is a 1960s Wild clampable mineral stage with interchangeable cork inserts; some idea of an extreme of its range is shown. To its right is an old live-box, which fits on to a microscope stage and allows the top plate to be slowly moved towards the bottom to trap the subject without injury. In front is a pair of free-standing cover glass forceps, normally closed, which are very useful to hold largish flat subjects. In front of those is another pair of normally closed forceps, as used in electrical assembly work, and useful also for supporting gently but firmly an assortment of subjects. In front of all the rest are two kinds of stage forceps. The wire cage on the left opens and closes to grip larger and smaller irregularly shaped subjects, while on the right conventional double-ended stage forceps have small normally closed forceps at one end, and a cork disc to take pins at the other. Both fit into a hole in an ordinary mechanical stage, and both rotate about their own axes as well as moving to and fro. This range of older equipment can be emulated in the workshop if original examples are not to be found second-hand; all are invaluable resources in reflected-light work in the macro range.

## 4.3 Supporting larger specimens

For focal lengths between about 80 mm and 120 mm, there is plenty of working distance to arrange lighting, and the specimens tend to require more levelling or tilting than more complicated arranging. A gliding stage is an asset for rapid gross positioning, and a few tiny wedges or blocks will be invaluable for angle adjustment, while carrying sometimes quite heavy loads without slowly yielding during exposure (*Figure 4.3*).

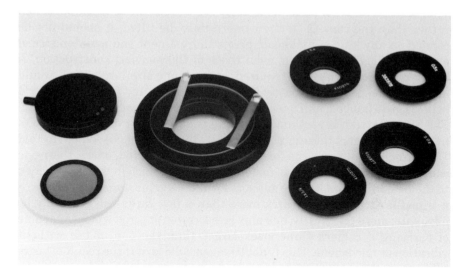

**Figure 4.3:** Wild gliding stage.
The Wild gliding stage fits the illuminating bases of their stereomicroscopes and macroscopes. It moves about 1 cm in each direction, and the ease of movement can be controlled using heavier or lighter grease between the sliding parts (lighter is used for easier movement to follow more rapidly moving organisms). Larger versions are easily made up in the workshop, and some rolling on individual ball bearings are possible for larger versions still. The standard glass disc can be replaced by that shown, carrying a polarizer. Also shown are the supplementary lenses of the M420, and the attachable rotatable quarter-wave plate. Top left is the attachable analyser, fitting over the lenses. Such equipment is usable with other makes of apparatus, of course.

## 4.4 The use of illuminating bases

The kind of bases supplied for use with stereo microscopes may provide combined support and illumination quite conveniently for smallish specimens. The lighting which goes with such bases is rarely sophisticated, and may be only two or three small focusing tungsten lamps carried on mobile arms and worked from a variable transformer in the base itself. Quite often the bases have sockets for attaching lamps, and these can be useful for using separate and possibly more adaptable lamps. Some bases allow transmitted illumination to be used at the same time as reflected, from the one transformer, and this can be helpful to control shadows, provided the two are separately controllable. In general, these bases provide routine illumination, and not the more sophisticated lighting needed for complex subjects.

## 4.5 Supporting the camera at special angles

This is best avoided if possible; rigidity is assured by tilting the specimen rather than the camera. If the camera must be tilted, it should not be carried on any kind of ball head; precise adjustment and maintenance of angle is difficult with these, even those of the heaviest construction. A heavy pan-and-tilt head is required, at least one size larger than would usually be needed for the particular camera in use, and two sizes larger if bellows are attached, or if a technical camera is in use at longer extension. The Sinar pattern is recommended, and is suitable for any camera up to half-plate format in these circumstances, while being small enough to hold 35 mm bellows. If a large-format camera is attached, more than one camera screw should be used, fastened to a plate which in turn is attached to the head (*Figure 4.4*). The support for the head must also be massive – a tripod far too heavy to carry more than a few yards will generally be adequate; more practically, one may be borrowed or hired which is capable of carrying a camera three sizes larger than the one in use without vibration or movement. This is not frivolous advice; it is the result of years

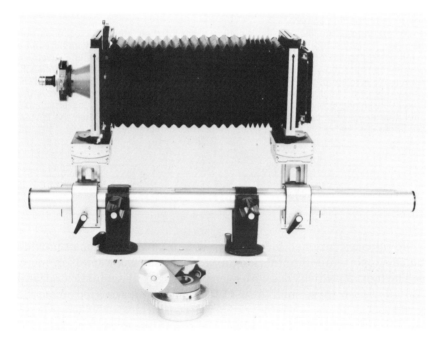

**Figure 4.4:** Camera mounted on two clamps.
Whether used vertically or horizontally, a camera at longer extension than usual should always have more than one support. The Sinar P shown has its extended rail carried on two clamps, carried in turn on a thick aluminium plate. This is attached to the Sinar pan-and-tilt head, resulting in an exceptionally rigid set-up. The same principles apply to all cameras, and such a plate is easily made up to any required length. A snout is attached to the lens plate, with a Compur Electronic 1 shutter.

of experience of using highly magnifying camera systems, which definitely require much better support than cameras working at infinity. Best of all is to attach the camera support to a heavy permanent framework but, as such camera angles are most often required away from the studio, recourse must be made to supports as described above. It is possible to make up such supports much more cheaply than heavy professional tripods can be purchased, of course; they do not have to look good, but they must be strong and rigid for the circumstances required. The usual technique of weighting ordinary tripods with sandbags slung from them or draped over them is also helpful in providing low-level weight and stability.

Some proprietary components may be useful for camera support, especially on location, if the camera is neither too heavy nor too long. The tubes in the Foba photographic-support system are heavy and rigid, with good clamps; those in the older Alpa Macrostat system are lighter but no less rigid, and with good baseclamps and mounts (*Figure 3.13*). Some lighter laboratory scaffold units (such as Climpex) might be used in some circumstances, if they are suitably erected with bracing. Comprehensive systems such as Macrostat include focusing stage components, ground-spikes, mirrors on flexible stems and more, and are especially useful if kept as a cased set for location work. Naturally, components from more than one system can be used in conjunction, and this is very often desirable.

# 4.6 Supporting living specimens

Different considerations apply to specimens in a horizontal dish or in a vertical aquarium. If the specimen is in the former (possibly using various sizes of plastic disposable Petri dishes, which are of high optical and mechanical quality), a gliding stage will allow movement to be followed for either still or motion pictures. A difficulty is that the background may possibly be obtrusive; if the dish is supported at a small distance over a piece of matt black velvet, reflections and shadows will be controlled effectively, and a darkground effect can then be obtained to enhance contrast. Other colours of matt velvet are obtainable for other effects; a light red velvet is effective if a blue lighting is used, giving an effect akin to Rheinberg illumination.

For vertical aquaria a support similar to that recommended for small specimens is needed if movement is to be followed, as it will usually be necessary to follow this in three planes. The illumination in such cases is best arranged by fibre optics supported to light the image area, so that the specimens are moved into it for constant lighting; a foot-controlled release for the shutter is usually an advantage in such case, as both hands are needed to operate stage controls.

A vertical aquarium can easily be made up as required, from large microscope slides joined by silicone rubber cement. This is tough but flexible and totally waterproof once set, and the glass is, of course, of the highest quality. It is often useful to arrange the front glass to be at a slight tilt to the vertical, to avoid reflections of the lens showing in it, especially if a darkground effect is obtained with the illumination (*Figure 4.5*). A further slide kept in place inside by small wedges will restrict the freedom of movement of the organisms to a suitable area. This is an old device, with wedges made from ivory in the nineteenth century; nowadays they are easily cut from polythene. A variety of miniature aquaria (vertical and horizontal) can be found in old microscopical outfits, and examples should always be acquired if offered. A variety of compressoria and liveboxes can

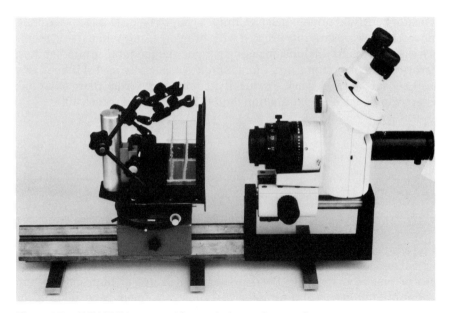

**Figure 4.5:** Wild M420 mounted for vertical aquarium work.
A student-type optical bench 0.25 m in length was mounted on a heavy common baseplate carrying a holder for the Wild M420 macroscope, and provided with outrigger feet shod with rubber. A long carrier was fitted with a rebuilt mechanical stage from a Russian metallurgical microscope, to provide rapid, coarse focusing (by sliding to and fro), and precise movement and rotation of the $x$ and $y$ axes. To the top plate of the stage was fitted part of the column of an old inverted Prior microscope, which carries a stage that can be easily adjusted vertically. In front is a mask of matt black Formica, against which is pushed an aquarium made from large microscope slides held together with silicone rubber cement. The front plate is slightly tilted so as to avoid reflections of the lens. To the rear of the stage are fitted small clamps to hold fibre-optic tungsten/flash focusing lightguides. Organisms under study are allowed to settle down in the aquarium for some hours at least, and are then found at low power and low light level. The stage is then adjusted in all axes to provide the required view, and the zoom and/or front lenses adjusted to provide the required magnification. In the figure no camera is attached, but a 35 mm body (or a larger format still camera or a video camera) can be used with its own relay tube to provide accurate focusing via the eyepieces. A foot-operated cable release is normal, if the stage controls have to be operated to follow an active organism, at magnifications of up to $\times 50$.

also be very useful for holding and controlling active organisms, and these also can still be found second-hand (*Figure 4.6*). Coloured backgrounds are easily arranged behind such an aquarium to provide suitable colour contrasts to the organisms being recorded, especially if these are being lit by fibre optics with colour filters in place.

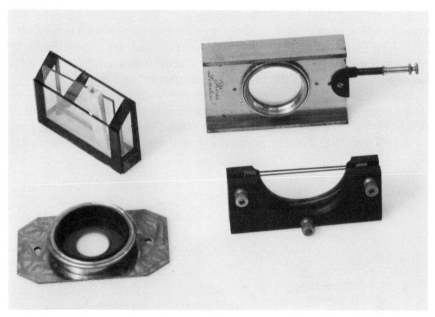

**Figure 4.6:** Aquaria for close-range work.
Top left is the classic glass aquarium of the nineteenth century, which is held together by marine glue, and which has an internal glass plate and ivory wedge to control the position of active organisms. Below this is a live-box that is used horizontally, suitable for wet specimens, and with a lid which can be lowered slowly just to hold an organism in place. Top right is a compressorium that uses slowly driven wedges to hold an organism; this pattern can be used vertically or horizontally and, as such, is especially versatile. In front on the right is a Botterill trough, consisting of two clamping-plates held together with screws which contain two standard microscope slides separated by part of a red rubber sealing ring for glass jars. This admirable demountable miniature aquarium works (with a very thin separator) horizontally or (with a thicker separator) vertically.

## 4.7 Working in field conditions

Such conditions presuppose a need to follow a free-living organism, frame it promptly, and expose immediately. A camera with suitable extension tubes is best for this, with proper macro lenses as opposed to mere close-focusing camera lenses. Using 35 mm single-lens cameras with though-the-lens (TTL) metering for flash for such purposes confers immense advantages, as they are lighter and more flexible than medium formats. It is possible to have as one rigid handleable unit the camera, tube and flash, and to expose using the eye-level viewfinder as usual. Few manufacturers make actual macro lenses specifically for this format, but one special exception is Olympus. Their two macro lenses of shortest focus (focal lengths of 20 mm and 38 mm) are in automatic-diaphragm bayonet mounts, and (as already mentioned) in addition to the usual extension tubes, Olympus make a telescopic version which gives a range of magnifications with one lens in place (*Figure 4.7*). The author adapted his Hasselblad 55 mm extension tube to have a spiral focus which extends its length steplessly to 90 mm, and such adaptations are not difficult to achieve in a good workshop. Add to such a unit dedicated flash and TTL flash exposure control off the film during exposure, and this forms a very versatile and high-quality hand-held unit.

Even with a reflex camera, it can be useful to use a frame instead of looking through the usual finder. For example, if a frame (perhaps purpose-made from a carefully bent metal coat-hanger wire, ideal in its

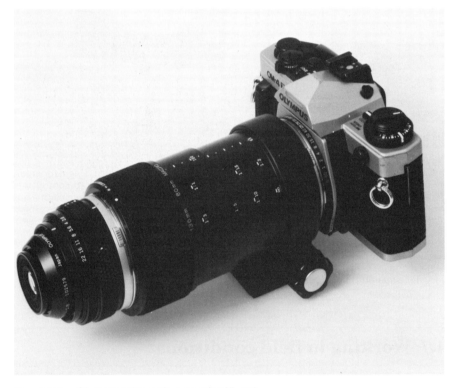

**Figure 4.7:**  Olympus telescopic auto tube 65–116.
This tube is often used in the field, as it varies in length from 65 to 116 mm, and locks at any extension in its range with a twist while maintaining automatic diaphragm action. It is shown fitted to an Olympus OM4Ti body, and carrying the Olympus 38 mm macro lens in auto-diaphragm mount. The tube is marked with magnification values for Olympus macro-range lenses. The author has modified a Hasselblad 55 extension tube to give multi-start spiral focusing action of a range between 55 and 90 mm, while maintaining automatic diaphragm action. Such tubes are most useful in the field.

characteristics for this purpose) is arranged to surround the precise image area at a particular focus setting of lens and tube combination, it can be much simpler to place the frame in the best plane round the subject while viewing gross from the side. The behaviour of the organism in its immediate surroundings is more easily viewed and predicted in this way than when looking at the organism (only) with the normal optical finder. This technique yields excellent results. It is equally applicable to medium formats, which are then held with mirror already raised, making for a smoother and quieter exposure. It is also applicable to even a $4 \times 5$ inch baseboard camera, previously set up via its ground-glass screen in just the same way (*Figure 4.8*). The results can be magnificent, provided one remembers to remove the darkslide cover before exposure!

If the luxury of using a tripod is possible in the field, in the particular circumstances of an assignment (not all organisms move quickly and/or unpredictably), the choice of the tripod itself is an important consideration. It should be waterproof (the legs of an ordinary tripod fill with water

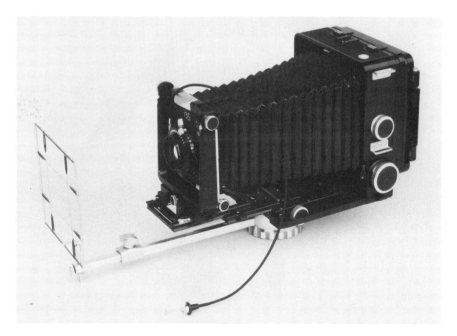

**Figure 4.8:** Wista $4 \times 5$ inch camera fitted with framing wires.
This is an old and sophisticated Linhof frame-finder, which is attached to the camera bush by an extendable arm that allows for height adjustment and that has movable framing wires on springs to keep them taut. The camera is supported with its extension giving the required magnification, and the framing wires are moved so as to be just outside the field of view when checked on the ground-glass screen. The lens aperture is then set, the flash attached if required, the shutter closed, the film back of whatever format attached, and the darkslide removed. Any subject now framed by the wires is in focus and fully covered by the format in use, so that releasing the shutter by a cable release (perhaps attached to a pistol grip) secures an accurate picture. Such a framing device can be made up from bent iron-wire coat-hangers simply enough and with little expense.

quite easily given the chance), usable at low level and with an overhang. The author has used the unique Benbo tripod for over 20 years for such work in 35 mm and, with care, for medium format also. This tripod can be used to support the camera in a wide variety of positions (e.g. close to a vertical wall) and is physically strong.

In all work with a tripod in the field, the use of a focusing slide to move the whole camera/bellows or camera/tubes system to and fro is a necessity. If such a piece of equipment is used, it must be large and very solid; many versions are on sale, but many are unsuitable (*Figure 4.9*). If a stand from an old type of microscope is available, the main body tube slideways can

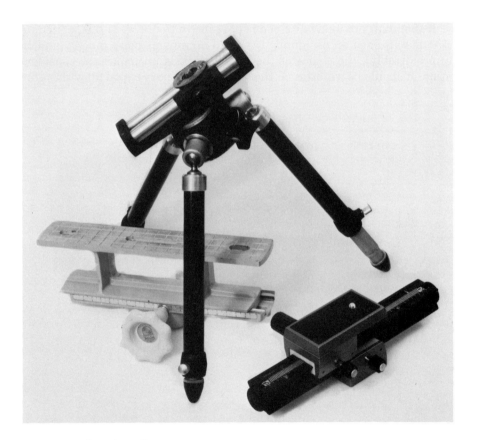

**Figure 4.9:** Focusing rails.
The Pentacon mini-tripod and clamping focusing rail is shown. They are suitable for 35 mm cameras which have to be supported at odd angles for reflected-light macro-range work. Each leg of the tripod moves in a full arc when the single clamping knob is loosened, and each leg also has an extension; together these offer a very wide range of support possibilities that are ideal for use in the field. The focusing rail has been modified to provide a lower attachment than the original, and the rails and clamping carrier are very rigid in use. In front is the Olympus focusing rail, with rack and pinion-driven clamping camera platform (suitable for 35 mm and 6 × 6 cm cameras) and rack and pinion-driven clamping focusing drive which attaches to the tripod or to a heavy-duty stand. The lighter-coloured Linhof clamping focusing rail is heavy duty, suitable for even 4 × 5 inch cameras, which can be attached as needed in several places on the top.

be removed and milled off to make a base for a camera attachment, to make an excellent rack-and-pinion focusing slide (with fine adjustment into the bargain if need be). The body tube is removed and a milled camera platform substituted, with the screw tightened from below. This adapter lacks only a clamping screw, and it is worth adding one in some way, so that the focus, once secured, does not imperceptibly alter (although some stands have built-in tightening to the coarse slideways). Any commercial focusing slide should have a clamping screw, and adequate ones are supplied by companies such as Nikon and Olympus (to fit their bellows units also). Slides moving in two planes are also available, but as these introduce a further source of potential unwanted motion, the author does not recommend them for magnifications much above × 2.

For all macro-range work on a tripod, it is strongly recommended (if circumstances permit) to set up the focus and then to pause for 3 or 4 sec with the apparatus untouched before making the exposure (using a cable release at least 500 mm long); this allows vibrations to die down.

## 4.8 Direct illumination methods

The choice and use of illumination methods is precisely the same as in ordinary photography, but on a small scale, and thus requiring much less power. The usual techniques of lighting for modelling, texture, contrast and effect are those described in photographic textbooks for product photography, portraiture, advertising and so forth, with some special considerations added (for lighting ideas, see Anstee, 1984; Carlson and Carlson, 1991; Giebelhausen and Althann, 1967; Marchesi, 1988). The basic choice is between tungsten (longer exposure) work and flash (shorter exposure) work. For reflected-light work, it is always an advantage if the lens is carried proud of the front of its camera on a snout, which allows higher-angled lighting units to act without obstruction.

Tungsten lighting may be used with great effect and control unless rapid movement of the image must be stopped. One largely used source is the separate microscope lamp, tungsten or tungsten–halogen, but these are now much less common than they were, with the advent of almost universal built-in illumination in compound microscopes. Their quality varies enormously, and a check should be made to see that a small spot can be focused close by. Such units tend to be quite small if they use a tungsten lamp, and larger if they use a tungsten–halogen lamp (*Figure 4.10*). As the two produce different colour temperatures they should not be mixed in any one shot if colour is in use. Although such units are generally mounted on rods above or separately from their transformer units, adjusting several of them to light one small subject can be tricky, as they tend to get in the way of each other if close by. They should be fitted individually with

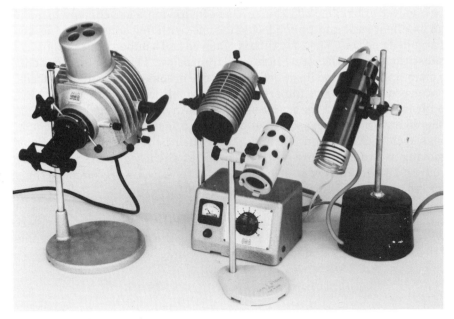

**Figure 4.10:** Microscope lamps.
These are becoming less common with the advent of stands having built-in illumination. On the left is the Wild Universal lamp, with well- ventilated large housing, a quartz collector lens, a throw-in ground-glass, and an iris with a long control lever. It is shown fitted with its plug-in filter carrier, which has an additional tilting interference filter holder. The housing takes centring holders for a 12V 100W tungsten–halogen lamp, or a high-pressure xenon or mercury arc, as required. The power unit is separate, as needed, allowing the lamp to be positioned closely to a subject needing a lot of light for its illumination. In the middle is the Wild lamphouse for a 6V 30W, tungsten lamp, in a centring holder, with a focusing collector lens and iris, and a double filter tray. It adjusts widely on its power-supply base. On the right is a Prior lamphouse with 6V 30W tungsten lamp in a centring focusing holder, with collector, iris and triple filter tray. The power supply is in the base, and the lamp is widely adjustable on its stand. In front is a more modern Russian lamp, also 6V 30W tungsten, with a focusing collector, iris and single filter tray. Its power supply is separate. Such a variety of lamps, some of which are no longer available, is valuable for lighting reflected-light subjects in macro-range work, and can often be found relatively cheaply second-hand nowadays.

heat-absorbing filters, for several of them lighting a small object with focused beams can produce a significant and damaging rise in its temperature. They are easy to fit with colour filters if different sides of an object need different colouring for a particular result. Some of them, such as the Wild Universal lamp, have quartz condensers which are useful for UV work.

A much better source is the fibre-optic lamp, which uses tungsten–halogen sources with dichroic filters to reduce the longer wavelength infrared heat content. (They are not the unit of choice for some infrared work with certain TV sensors as a result, although they pass shorter wavelength infrared for use with special film.) The illumination is carried along shorter or longer fibres, with lenses at the end of the bundle to focus the light into quite a tight spot. The ends can be rigid and self-supporting, and they do stay in place for long periods (*Figure 4.11*). Some larger

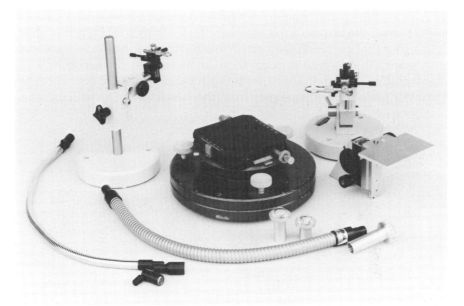

**Figure 4.11:** Supports and fibre-optics for reflected-light work.
In the centre is the heavy levelling base holding a Russian mechanical stage from a metallurgical stand. This is excellent for positioning small objects for macro-range work, and is immovable in use. Also shown are two current Prior supports for micromanipulation, ideal for precise positioning of some objects for reflected-light work. A further Prior stand has been modified to take a small stage for vertical adjustment, with both coarse and fine focusing incorporated; it attaches to the stage on a heavy base to give precise orientation in all three planes. A standard lightguide is also shown with the usual focusing lens; a wide-diameter guide (with much greater light-carrying capacity) and a homemade focusing carrier for a moulded plastic aspheric lens, which can be bought quite cheaply, can also be seen.

bundles need end support, but do carry a lot more of the light. The bundles can be single, or one might bifurcate to give two equal beams distally, or a bundle might illuminate a ring (by a continuous circle or by four separate outlets). This last unit has much potential: used above the subject it will give nearly shadowless lighting; used below (at the right distance) it will give a darkground or rim-lit effect. Filters can be inserted into the body of the unit to affect all the output, and there is usually control of the brightness, often without affecting the colour temperature; this allows several units to be used in combination while varying the effect. The colour temperature of the lamps allows tungsten–halogen microscope lamps to be used with them, to give limitless combinations of effect.

The result of using such lamps is to give harsh shadows and much contrast in the image. Stray light can easily affect the overall result, and the use of pieces of matt black velvet round the illuminated area, and especially in front of the limb or pillar of the stand, is a wise precaution. A beam arranged for grazing illumination (horizontally across the top of the specimen) is a good start in setting up; merely lowering the source a little will give rim lighting, or raising it will soften shadows. A more pronounced light will usually be needed from one direction (the key light), to give moulding and roundness. After that, adjustment and careful inspection on the screen of the camera will slowly progress towards ideal lighting for that particular subject. While having the subject in place and ideally angled, it is good practice to make more than one exposure with slightly different illuminations, for it is difficult to judge the final effect on a print or projected transparency from the viewfinder of a small camera.

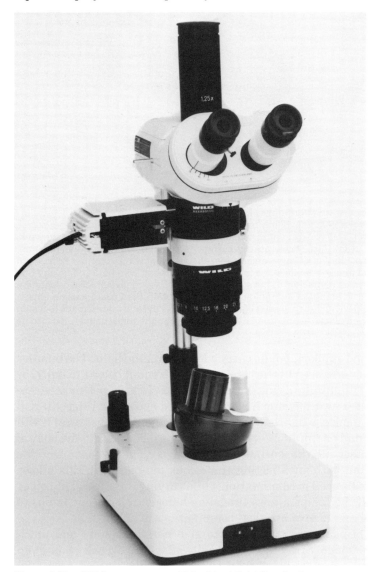

**Figure 4.12:** Wild macroscope with incident-light illuminator.

This accessory attaches rapidly and easily, to provide truly axial, incident, high-intensity illumination. It is shown with the stand carrying the cup-stage, which allows tilt in the optical axis. The tube shown on the stage was perfectly illuminated at a depth of 2 cm, which is difficult to achieve in other ways. Smaller versions of the stage can be made up using half a ping-pong ball filled with plaster of Paris and loaded with a dark or suitably coloured pigment.

With large-format cameras, this is less necessary, as a distant view of the whole screen gives an adequate impression of the final result.

A special tungsten unit for the Wild macroscope is available, attaching behind the lens unit, and providing excellent axial illumination through the lens (*Figure 4.12*). This is invaluable for a general basic light, and more so for illuminating cavities. For almost the same effect, Nikon supply Lieberkühns and semi-reflecting vertical illuminators for two of their macro lenses. The Lieberkühns are used on the transmitted-light base, of course, but the vertical illuminators can be used with any separate light source wherever is convenient (*Figure 4.13*). These items are expensive, but can be more than worth it. Second-hand Lieberkühns are not infrequently found and, if their focal lengths are right, are easily adapted to modern low-power objectives. Lieberkühns can be simulated using aluminium cooking foil, moulded to an approximate focus, or an old torch reflector. An axial illuminator can sometimes be simulated using a suitably sized coverglass fixed to the front of a lens at 45° by Blu-tack™.

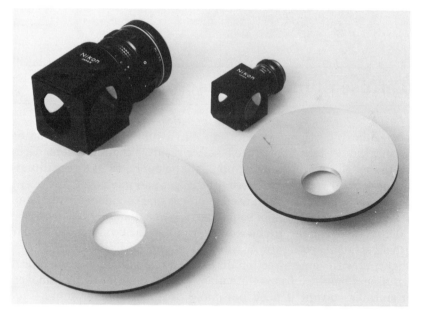

**Figure 4.13:** Nikon Lieberkühns and vertical illuminators.
An especially valuable feature of the Nikon macro-dia equipment is its provision of Lieberkühns and vertical illuminators for two of their macro lenses, the 35 mm and 65 mm. The Lieberkühns attach above the lens to receive illumination around the subject resting on the transmitted-light base before focusing it back; this achieves virtually shadowless lighting. Similar, but smaller, devices were very popular in the nineteenth century for use with objectives of focal lengths as short as 0.5 inch. The vertical illuminators need not be used on the illuminating base, of course, as they receive their light from the side from any suitable lamp, directing some of it through the lens to the subject for true vertical illumination and receiving it back to form the image. Such devices were also much used as accessories, until recently, for shorter focal lengths altogether.

With flash, it is much more difficult to visualize the final result unless the units have modelling lamps incorporated, and few which are suitable for macro-range work have these. In the past, Bowens produced units specifically for low-power macro-range work, as do Olympus, but nowadays the best recommendation that can be made is to have fibre-optic lamphousings which incorporate flash units. These give the best of both worlds, and it is possible to work a flash-head through a fibre-optic source-housing; all that is needed is a large coverglass reflector mounted at 45° inside the housing, in front of the lamp. An opening in the top of the housing can then accept any suitably powered and smallish head (perhaps held in place only with Blu-tack™ or the like); the positioning is not unduly critical. The tungsten now serves only as a modelling light, and with off-the-film (OTF) flash control in the camera, macro-range work with active organisms is greatly facilitated. A commercial version of this apparatus, the Novoflex 'Macrolight Plus', is now available (from Fotogerätebau K. Müller, see Appendix). Flash remains the illuminant of choice, of course, for all actively moving subjects, and every effort must be made to visualize the results if no modelling lights are included in the system, since the short duration of the exposure and its lack of heat are more important attributes than its drawbacks in such cases.

# 4.9 Diffuse illumination methods

Where specular reflections are a nuisance in a subject, recourse must be had to some kind of tent to produce a softer result, but similar considerations as to modelling and showing-up of shape apply, as in direct illumination, and similar sources are used. For larger specimens, a translucent moulded lampshade (of the kind used in offices and corridors for tungsten lamps) forms a seamless tent of some merit with a diameter between 100 and 200 mm; these can be purchased in various sizes and shapes and their use with directional spotlights, possibly on a light-box base also, produces a soft lighting with some directionality. Modern small circular or conical food containers moulded from white plastic (with their lettering removed with a suitable solvent if need be) make excellent smaller tents (*Figure 4.14*). Failing such a shade, a thin sheet of translucent plastic can be made into a cone of suitable height and shape; keep the overlap small or it will show as a line in the result. At a pinch, or for less diffusion, a sheet of greaseproof paper will serve similarly, if the cone is not too large (although the cone should, in all cases, be quite noticeably larger than the subject).

For small specimens a tiny tent may be contrived from two-thirds of a ping-pong ball or from two-thirds of the shell of a boiled egg (*Figure 4.15*); in these cases the specimen rests on the bottom of the tent, often held by

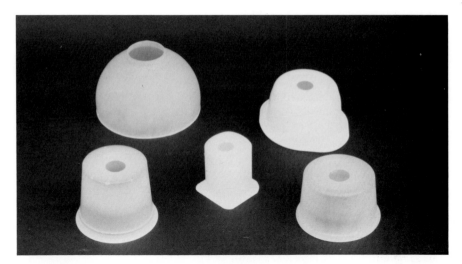

**Figure 4.14:** Tents for shadowless illumination.

The figure shows a selection of plastic food containers of varying degrees of translucency, shape and size, with holes to allow access for the lens. On the top left is a ground-glass lamp shade, which is excellent if one can be found. Larger tents, if needed, also may be found in lighting departments, such as plastic lampshades for office use. A selection is very useful to keep to hand when recording objects with shiny surfaces.

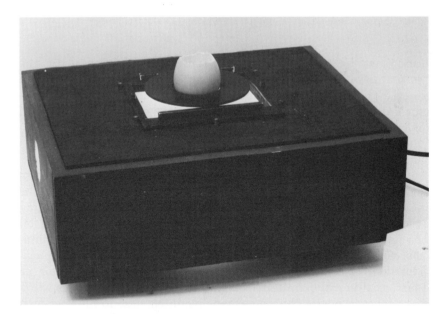

**Figure 4.15:** Small tent on light box.

The light box is lit, via a dimmer, by small mains-voltage tungsten filament lamps, giving even lighting and being suitable (with a 50-mired bluish filter) for tungsten film. On top, the shell of a boiled egg acts as a small tent for recording a tiny reflecting subject resting at the bottom. The (white) egg is soft-boiled, cooled, its top is cut off smartly with a heavy sharp knife, and the contents are spooned out to leave a perfect tiny tent. Illumination by the light-box alone, as with other kinds of tent, may be best, or extra lamps can be used to give some directionality.

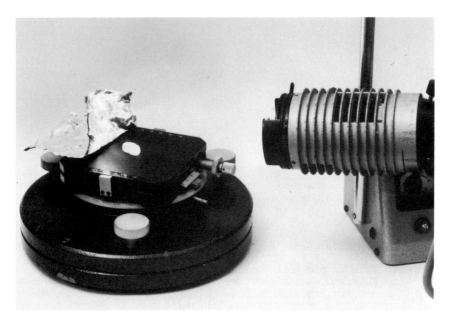

**Figure 4.16:**   Aluminium foil reflector.
On the macro stage, aluminium cooking foil can be used as a versatile reflector. It is used double or quadruple (to give some rigidity) and can actually be moulded to reflect the light as required (perhaps around a ping-pong ball), which is a helpful characteristic.

Blu-tack™, while the lens looks in at the top. The requirement is that the tent is seamless so as not to introduce markings on the surface of the specimen. For an approach to shadowless lighting, a macro ring illuminator (such as the old Leitz tungsten model mentioned in Section 3.8) or a current electronic ringflash are good starting points.

If the camera lens is tightly fitted with a white card, and similar cards are placed round the specimen so as to cover bright parts of the equipment, this may well suffice to control reflections, in emulation of white-room conventional studio photography. Use of slight lateral movement on the lens standard of a suitable camera may also be very helpful in eliminating reflections. To give some directionality to lighting, aluminium cooking foil may be set at one side, and moulded as required to reflect some illumination more or less actually at a focus on the subject; this has wide applicability for small objects (*Figure 4.16*). If available, a silver side-reflector (as used historically) will definitely focus illumination in this way, as will a substage concave mirror that is perhaps mounted close to the specimen (*Figure 4.17*).

A notorious case of unwanted reflections arises when material in small test-tubes or capillary tubes must be photographed. To counter such reflections they are best suspended in water contained in a flat-fronted water tank or aquarium made up specially as described under supporting living specimens (Section 4.6). If the face of the container is set at a slight

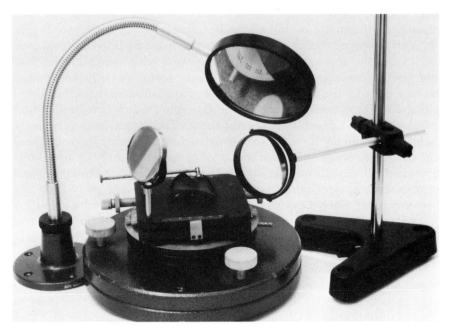

**Figure 4.17:** Reflectors for close-range work.
The macro stage carries holes to attach various accessories. Those shown are a silvered side-reflector (from about 1880), which fits round the macro lens to reflect focused light on to one side of the specimen from close range. Two ordinary substage mirrors are shown, one on a spacer carried direct by the stage, and a larger one on a stalk carried on a stand and clamp. A larger mirror still is shown attached to a flexible arm carried on a socket attachable to a baseboard (or to a ground-spike for outdoor use). The substage mirrors are double-sided, and can be used concave for focused lighting, or plane for less directional. (No camera is shown, to avoid confusion.)

angle to the lens, to avoid a reflection of the lens being recorded, little difficulty will then be experienced in lighting and recording the specimens. Such immersion is a possible technique for other objects, of course. Depending on the nature of a specimen, liquids other than water can be used – glycerol and cedar oil are possible, among others. Some increased depth of field is a further advantage of this method.

# 4.10 Illumination using a thin sheet of light

This treatment suits specimens of a particular shape only, where depth of field is otherwise grossly inadequate. The principle is that lighting from lamps at each side of the specimen is focused through narrow horizontal slits (which must not exceed in depth the depth of field of the lens as used), and the specimen is driven up along the optical axis through the resulting sheet of light. There are several variables – rate of ascent, depth of slits, intensity of illumination – but all can be combined with experience to give a properly exposed record of every layer of a deep specimen built-up over time to give the appearance of a single exposure with impossible depth of field. Only static subjects can be recorded in this way, and only those where the base is wider than the top. This kind of apparatus (patented in 1968) is available commercially, such as the Dynaphot which is manufactured by Irvine Optical Corporation (see Appendix). This is costly and very nicely made, but similar equipment can be constructed in the workshop, provided that the rising stage is smooth and precise in action and has no lateral movement (Clarke, 1993; Root, 1991). The apparatus is used in a darkened room, of course, and light must not be allowed to spill away from the specimen itself. Such a device is usable at magnifications from about × 5 to about × 100, given suitably supported specimens, and the results in terms of depth of field realized compared with conventional photomacrography are dramatic.

Much has been made in this chapter of the difficulties of supporting the subject and arranging its lighting. These are the keys to success, and time spent getting them just right is always time well spent. Further general notes on illumination in Chapter 5 should be read in conjunction with this chapter.

# References

**Anstee PT.** (1984) Light sources for photography. In *Photography for the Scientist* (2nd Edn) (ed. RA Morton). Academic Press, London.

**Beck R.** (1865) *A Treatise on the Construction, Proper Use . . . Achromatic Microscopes* (Reprinted in facsimile, Chicago: Science Heritage, 1987). Van Voorst, London.

**Carlson C, Carlson SE.** (1991). *Professional Lighting Handbook* (2nd Edn). Focal Press, London.

**Carpenter WB.** (1901) *The Microscope and its Revelations* (8th Edn, revised by WH Dallinger). Churchill, London.

**Clarke TM.** (1993) Image field size limitation for scanning light photomacrography. *The Microscope* **41**, 21–30.

**Croy OR.** (1961) *Camera Close Up*. Focal Press, London.

**Giebelhausen J, Althann H.** (1967) *Large Format Photography*. Grossbild Technik, Munich.

**Marchesi JJ.** (1988) *Professional Lighting Technique*. Verlag Photographie, Allschwil.

**Root N.** (1991) A simplified unit for making deep-field (scanning) macrographs. *J. Biol. Photography* **59**, 3–8.

# 5 General Remarks on Illumination and Exposure

## 5.1 Tungsten versus flash

The gist of the merits of each have been touched on in Chapter 4. Continuous illumination by tungsten has advantages in controlling contrast and direction of lighting (see Section 5.2), in addition to allowing clear visualization of the result, but very short-duration exposures (often needed with living organisms) are almost impossible to obtain. Flash illumination is often difficult to apply with visualization of the result, but applies little total heat to the subject and can last a few milliseconds only. Flash with modelling lights may be seen as an ideal, as it has in ordinary photographic studio work for many years; the author's personal preference remains with tungsten (for both), unless a short exposure is vital for the work in hand. Some general sources on photographic illumination should be consulted by the reader who may be inexperienced in commercial photography (see Anstee, 1984; Carlson and Carlson, 1991; Giebelhausen and Althann, 1967; Marchesi, 1988).

## 5.2 Split and multiple exposures

Exposures need not be given in one continuum, but in reflected-light work may often be split with great advantage. If the total length of tungsten exposure required was 10 sec, for example, then 6 sec could be given from one direction and 4 sec from another (perhaps grazing illumination, for example), using whatever light source was to hand. Similarly, if 6 sec of illumination was given under a tent, and 4 sec direct, then a more informative effect might be obtained than with tent or direct illumination alone. Use of the longest focal length of photographing lens possible gives sufficient working distance to allow removal of a tent between exposure times.

This is the basis of splitting exposures, and can also be used with flash, if, of course, the subject is static. Firing three flashes from one direction and two from another, for example, will allow lower-powered units to be used as well as giving a better quality of illumination. With both light sources, it may be well to avoid recocking the shutter for split exposures to avoid any movement at all of the image on the film; the use of a piece of card of suitable size covered with matt black velvet (on a handle or not, as required) held close below the lens but not touching it, while the lamp is moved and/or the flash recharges, gives perfect control without disturbing the set-up. This is, of course, exactly the same technique that is so useful to the architectural photographer when someone walks in front of his camera during a long exposure in a dark cathedral! Opportunity can be taken to use different colour filters over the lamps if contrast is to be given by this means, but this will certainly require the use of an assistant.

With tungsten lighting, one or more lamps can also be moved about during a longish exposure, softening the effect and giving a surprising amount of control. Movement in an arc in the vertical and/or the horizontal plane is very helpful in controlling excess contrast, especially when only one lamp is available; dwelling in one place gives greater final brightness from that direction, of course. This procedure is one well worth applying, in my experience.

Multiple exposures, putting several images on one frame, can also be useful, just as in normal-scale photography. This needs special care in the macro range, and often requires a mechanical stage (preferably driven by a stepping motor) or, perhaps more effectively still, a driven tilting stage. With 35 mm reflex cameras (allowing for checking of the focus and effect) and OTF quick-recharging electronic flash, very helpful records even of living organisms can be obtained. Darkground illumination is usually a requirement for success.

## 5.3 Colour temperature

As will be noted when considering colour films in more detail (Chapter 7), light sources based on both tungsten and flash exhibit a characteristic colour temperature. This is a measure of the blueness or redness of the illumination, with a theoretical basis in its equivalence to that emitted by a physicist's black body raised to a particular temperature measured in degrees Kelvin: the higher this temperature, the bluer the light. In practice, the main actual use of this concept is to allow sources to be balanced among themselves, and also to suit a particular emulsion. For that reason, the values are given in mireds (micro-reciprocal degrees; i.e. 10 000°K = 100 mireds, 4000°K = 250 mireds, 2500°K = 400 mireds, and so on) filters using these values have a constant effect on the blueness or redness of a source. Use of the scale bar (*Figure 5.1*) shows, for example, that a 6 V tungsten lamp has to be run at no less than 9 V to raise its colour

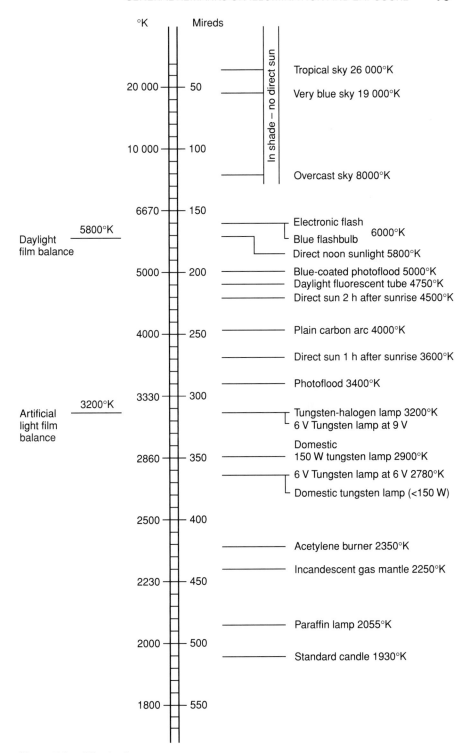

**Figure 5.1:** Mired values.

temperature to match a tungsten-balanced colour emulsion, while the same effect can be obtained (with much longer lamp life and production of much less heat) by using a bluish 50 mired filter over the lamp.

Series of colour-balancing filters with definite mired values are made by several companies, in gelatin, resin or glass, and are widely available. Brownish filters (to lower the colour temperature) might have a plus sign in front of their value, while bluish ones to raise the temperature might have a minus sign. If used for long periods over intense sources, it is as well to check them from time to time for fading.

## 5.4 Colour filters

The ordinary colour filters as used in general microscopy have the same place in macro-range work. They are used in transmitted-light work to control contrast, and the usual rule of choosing a filter from the other end of the spectrum to increase the contrast of a particular colour, and from the same end to reduce it and increase the rendering of detail, is equally valid. A blue filter is used to increase contrast in a red-stained specimen, and to increase detail in a blue-stained, for example (Bradbury, 1985). Similarly, a green filter increases contrast in a specimen coloured both blue and red, as a section stained with haematoxylin and eosin. It should be borne in mind that ordinary dyed filters may transmit a much wider range of wavelengths than is visually apparent, giving odd colour effects on some photographs. If they are to hand, suitable interference filters are to be preferred as their transmission has a much smaller bandwidth.

Some monochrome macro-range work in the nearer infrared is useful on occasion. For this, special emulsions are needed (see Chapter 6), together with a deep red filter for focusing, and a visually opaque one (passing none of the shorter wavelengths to which the film is also sensitive) for the actual exposure.

Infrared (heat) absorbing filters are needed over high-intensity lamps (see Section 5.5), and with some sources UV absorbing filters should also be used. High-wattage tungsten–halogen sources often need both; leaving excess UV in the illumination can give blurred images, as most emulsions are sensitive to the wavelengths transmitted by glass lenses.

## 5.5 Physical temperature

Intense illumination is required in reflected-light macrography at higher magnifications. It is easy to allow the physical temperature of specimens to be raised detrimentally while satisfactory illumination is being set up, which may take a long time. For this reason heat-absorbing filters should always be in place, although if fibre-optic sources are used, less heat is transmitted than with conventional lamps.

## 5.6 Misting

Control of contrast is often required in reflected-light work, and the use of tents has been advocated in Section 4.9 to minimize specular reflections. It is also worth considering cooling a suitable specimen once it has been set up, so that it will form a surface on which moisture from the air will condense for a few seconds; this achieves much the same effect as that used by the commercial photographer who sprays silverware with milk before photographing it! All that is needed is a gentle blast (so as not to overcool the specimen) from an aerosol of refrigerant (as used in histology and electronics). All should be ready when the dulling film of moisture appears (as if by magic) so that the exposure is made before the moisture evaporates again after a few seconds. Of course, a split exposure could record both the dulled and (soon afterwards) the undulled specimen to obtain just the required effect. This technique perhaps sounds unlikely, but it has given excellent effects in the hands of the author when all else has failed on account of the brightness and irregularity of the small object being pictured.

## 5.7 Additional material in the image plane

Mention has been made already of the use of drawing tubes with lowest-power objectives on the compound microscope, and that it is possible to introduce data such as clock-faces and graphics into the image plane. If such details are back-lit *and precisely masked off so that no glare is introduced into the primary image plane* with them, then proper control of the relative brightnesses of the two images will allow superimposition as required, cheaply and effectively. It is also possible to combine two separate images in this way, although this tends towards special-effects photography rather than proper scientific work.

## References

**Anstee PT.** (1984) Light sources for photography. In *Photography for the Scientist* (2nd Edn) (ed. RA Morton). Academic Press, London.

**Bradbury S.** (1985) Filters in microscopy. *Proc. R. Microsc. Soc.* **20**, 83–91.

**Carlson V and Carlson SE.** (1991) *Professional Lighting Handbook* (2nd Edn). Focal Press, London.

**Giebelhousen J and Anthann H.** (1967) *Large Format Photography.* Grossbild Technik, Munich.

**Marchesi JJ.** (1988) *Professional Lighting Technique.* Verlag Photographie, Allschwil.

# 6 Estimating Exposure in Macro-range Photography

## 6.1 TTL metering for transmitted light

With the now universal availability of TTL metering for both tungsten and flash exposures, the need to set down all that used to have to be said about exposure estimation has largely disappeared. TTL metering is the only choice for serious work in macro-range photography; that is, measuring the light intensity in the plane of the film itself. In some 35 mm cameras this is done for longer exposures by directing part of the image-forming rays on to a conjugate plane having a photoreceptor of one kind or another, and controlling the shutter speed under the actual conditions of intensity, aperture and extension obtaining. Exposures as long as several minutes can be automatically obtained by this means, the shutter closing when enough light has passed. For flash exposures the measurement is OTF; light reaches a receptor during the exposure, and when enough has been registered the flash is quenched.

Medium-format roll-film cameras can have similar devices built into their viewfinders, and for large-format cameras also a device such as the Sinarsix probe measures exposures, both for flash and for tungsten, in the film plane before an exposure is made. This is a slower process than for smaller cameras as it must be done before the darkslide is inserted, but it is equally valid for formats up to $10 \times 8$ inches.

## 6.2 Controlling TTL metering

All this is to the good, but some precautions are needed to ensure that one exposure, and one only, is required for any particular record. In transmitted-light work, the foolproof procedure is to take a reading of the clear background only, and to base the exposure on that (see Section 6.6). This ensures that it is this background brightness which is used as the reference level to determine the density of the final film. This is based on the fact that the brightness range in a transmitted-light picture in micro or macro

**79**

work can always be accommodated in the range accepted by all films used for such work. What is wanted is a background brightness one level of density higher than pure white in the final print (i.e. 0.1 D above background fog level in a monochrome film), and similarly in a colour transparency film. The sensors used in various cameras vary in colour sensitivity, but if they only ever measure background white light this will never matter. Further, the background is the brightest part of the image, and should be measurable even if it is rather dim. If the camera has a spot-reading facility, the spot is centred on an area of background (perhaps by moving the specimen), and the reading taken to give one unequivocal value, the meaning of which has been previously determined by calibration. It should be noted here that some cameras have their spot sensors fitted in such a way that they are affected by adjacent different brightnesses, and thus a large area of background only should be measured. If the camera does not have spot metering, the specimen may be moved bodily aside until only the background shows. With the Sinarsix meter on large format, the probe is simply moved to an area of background (so it is impossible to forget to return the specimen to centre-stage).

For transmitted illumination of other kinds, mainly darkground and polarizing in the macro ranges, separate calibration is carried out with them again using the background brightness only. Once this has been done, the method is used as above, and always provides unequivocal results.

When automatic units are used, such the Photautomat with the Wild M400 series, measurement can still be based on background readings, if they are made with the specimen moved aside, but the usual integrated readings can also be used if the unit is calibrated in advance, as described in Section 6.6.

## 6.3　TTL metering for reflected light

Integrated TTL measuring is needed for reflected-light exposure determination. If a tiny standard grey card can be held in the image plane, all well and good, and this should be read to obtain one definite value, calibrated in advance. If not, and providing reasonably balanced illumination has been set up, an integrated reading and automatic exposure will probably prove adequate. As such internal meters are adjusted to read a scene which approximates to a grey card in reflecting about 18% of the light reaching it, all will be well if this is about the level of reflectance of the macro object as lit. There is no substitute for experience in such work, and this may suggest an occasional lengthened or shortened exposure time for a particular set-up. If such experience is lacking, this is one of the very few situations in photography where the use of a short series of bracketed exposures would be recommended. The time taken to arrange the average macro set-up is so long that the use of a few extra frames in obtaining a satisfactory negative is fully justified.

For large formats, the Sinarsix is used in a similar manner, but perhaps more easily. With a larger screen it is sometimes possible to place the probe on the image of an area of the subject which has about 18% reflectance, and this provides one definite reading. It is also possible to use Polaroid material to make a quick trial exposure, allowing for any difference in speed of the materials; the expense of this may be justified in such a case.

## 6.4 Other kinds of metering for transmitted light

If the camera which must be used does not have TTL metering, the brightness of its screen (of whatever size) may be measurable by placing a fibre-optic probe light meter against it, such as the Profi-flex attached to the Gossen Mastersix, which measures a circle of diameter 5 mm (*Figure 6.1*); again, measuring the background only is strongly recommended here. Similarly, a spot meter (with acceptance angle of 1°) may be used to measure one definite background area of the screen, as before; this will have to be done at some distance from it unless a supplementary lens is attached. If so, as the one definite reading of background brightness is all that is needed, and if the meter is always used for such work with a particular lens attached, no special account of it need be taken. The Pentax spot meter (using a silicon photo diode) has a 20-stop measuring range, accurate to one-third of a stop, ample for such a purpose. The classic SEI Photometer remains totally serviceable in this kind of use; it has a range of 1 000 000 : 1, an acceptance angle of 0.5°, and a low cost on the second-hand market. Some spot meters, such as the Minolta Spotmeter F (with a range of 22.5 stops), have flash measurement capability also, and all that is needed is a series of trial flash exposures against a reading of the background brightness on the screen to choose the best exposure and thus to set the flash equipment output for the future. In all such cases, no difficulty will be experienced in obtaining unequivocal readings, to be interpreted against prior calibration.

## 6.5 Other kinds of metering for reflected light

The meters mentioned in Section 6.4 are also useful for reflected-light work. The fibre-optic probe will be small enough to be held above some

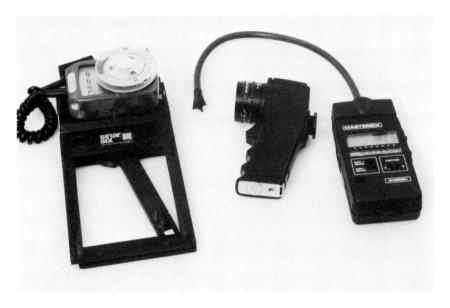

**Figure 6.1:**   Exposure meters.
On the left is the Sinarsix meter, which puts the sensor into the image plane; the area measured is shown by the small light rectangle on the probe, and it is obvious that selective readings are very easy to make. In the middle is a Pentax spot meter, which will take a 1° reading from a distance. On the right is the Mastersix meter with a fibre-optic probe attached, which has a 5 mm diameter reading spot. All of these are helpful if the camera being used has no TTL exposure-reading facility.

objects to get a camera-eye view of the set-up as lit so that the average brightness can be determined from close by; such results are easily calibrated for absolute values, taking into account bellows length and aperture settings as required. The spot meters are almost always usable for reflected-light work, working from a distance and perhaps with a supplementary lens to obtain a reading from the most significant part of the object (in exposure terms) to be used as the basis of exposure estimation. It may be possible on larger cameras to take out both the lens panel and focusing screen, to allow a meter to measure along the optical axis. A factor has to be used in such a case to allow for the effect on the aperture of the camera extension in use. The *effective f*-number is:

$$vf/F = f(m + 1),$$

where $v$ = lens-to-image distance, $f$ = marked $f$ number, $F$ = focal length of the lens, and m = magnification.

The big difference between TTL metering of whatever kind and non-TTL metering is that the former automatically corrects for bellows extension and aperture selected, whereas non-TTL metering requires various factors to be applied to the raw reading in order to arrive at the true reading, thus taking time and making room for error. Flash photography may be assisted by using the nomogram in *Figure 6.2*.

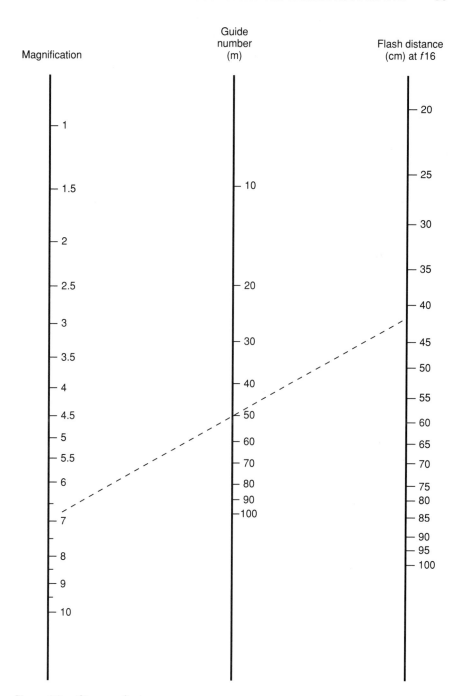

**Figure 6.2:**   Close-up flash nomogram.

Wherever filters of any density are to be applied, it is always best to read the exposure with white light, and then to introduce the filter and multiply by its experimentally determined factor (which might be surprisingly high). This avoids difficulties with an overall lack of sensitivity in the meter, or differential sensitivity to different colours.

## 6.6 Calibrating equipment

Whatever meters are used, the system must be calibrated experimentally, once and for all, against readings obtained when specific films are exposed and particular processing adopted. The basis is that a series of exposure times is used for each of several readings with the metering equipment, for each film and processing combination. The results are evaluated in the case of negatives first by inspection and then by actually printing the chosen negative (colour or monochrome); the measured value that gives the best result is the value to be adopted in future. For colour transparencies, evaluation is by actual projection to determine the value to be applied in future (unless large formats are in use, when inspection on a bright daylight viewing box is used).

A suitable median film speed is selected, and three exposures made each side of it at half-stop intervals (an accuracy of a half-stop is required for best final results). If a 35 mm camera is used, full frames are exposed; if roll film or sheet film is used, the slide is partly withdrawn and three exposures are made on one sheet. It is, of course, possible to make more, but if this is done the area available for evaluation is likely to be too small. The prescribed processing conditions (see Chapter 7) should be adhered to *rigorously*, and the best frame chosen. In this context, the best negative frame is that which has median density and produces a full range of tones on medium-contrast paper, and the best transparency is that which has a background just short of fully transparent (or of correct density if made by DIC or darkground illumination) when viewed over a proper light box.

If the camera is one with an automatic setting of the film speed (DX-coded films) it should have a knob which allows film speed to be adjusted within a range of 2 stops. If it does not have this facility, put black tape over the squares on the cassette (to stop it giving a reading), and set the speeds manually over the required range. If you cannot do this with the camera in use, change the camera. Automatic equipment is used for calibration simply by setting a range of film speeds.

Once this calibration has been carried out for each film and developer combination, and if need be for each type of illumination in use, vast amounts of time and materials will be saved. It is a chore, but it is one of the most worthwhile chores in this kind of photography. One value as read by whatever kind of meter is in use will give one exposure time, and one exposure only need then be given.

It cannot be stressed too forcefully that keeping full records, *made at the time*, of the several variables in both calibration and ordinary work will repay the tedious writing involved many times over. Sooner or later a difficulty will be encountered which may well be solvable by referring to proper records of what has already been done at some time in the past, and a great deal of time can be saved if the effort is made routinely to keep proper, rigorous records. Having to hand a studio record book, and a pen to use with it, are prerequisites.

# 7  Recording the Image

## 7.1  A survey of image-recording processes

A surprising number of imaging technologies exist today, although many
of them are for highly specialized purposes only. They can be summarized
as follows.

1. Graphic processes: require an artist who may work from the original
   image (with or without mechanical aids) in line, air-brush, scraper-
   board, water-colour or oil-colours and others; reproduced by lithogra-
   phy, gravure, letterpress, screen-printing or ink-jet systems.
2. Silver halide imaging: in monochrome or colour, chromogenic or not.
3. Chemical imaging: thermal, dye-imaging, photopolymer, or diazo.
4. Electronic imaging: television, video monitors for radar and medical
   purposes, computer-generated pictures.
5. Electrophotographic imaging: electrostatic, xerography.

The above list is far from complete, but shows the range to be very widely
based.

### 7.1.1  Criteria for assessing the behaviour of imaging systems

A wide variety of aspects of a system can be used to assess its suitability
for particular purposes.

1. Does it image in real time, or is access delayed?
2. What is the sensitivity of the receptor?
3. What is its nature and wavelength response?
4. Is a latent image formed, and is it stable?
5. How great an amplification does the system yield?
6. What is the nature of any noise recorded?
7. What is the nature of the final image and what is its level of digitiza-
   tion?
8. What is its modulation transfer function (see Ray, 1994)?
9. What is the stability of the final image?

Question 2, for example, might consider some of the details given in *Table 7.1*.

Answers to many of the questions on criteria may be difficult to obtain. For additional photographic information see Langford, 1986, 1989; Morton, 1984; Ray, 1983, 1994; Stroebel *et al.*, 1990.

**Table 7.1:**  Sensitivity of imaging systems

| Type of system | ASA speed (median) | Exposure required in lux (for lux-sec at 1/60 sec) | Photons/pixel or grain area/cm$^2$ |
|---|---|---|---|
| Photopolymer | 0.001 | 48 000 | $3 \times 10^{14}$ |
| Xerography | 1 | 48 | $3 \times 10^{11}$ |
| Silver halide | 100 | 0.48 | $3 \times 10^{9}$ |
| Electronic | 10 000 | 0.0048 | $3 \times 10^{7}$ |

# 7.2 Graphics processes

Drawing a microscopical image was for a long time the only way to record it, but nowadays this is only done occasionally. The advantages of a graphical record are compelling: one picture can be synthesized from a larger number; several image planes can be recorded together even if they were not all in focus together originally; confusing detail can be omitted; particular features can be emphasized; and the picture can carry clear labels. In short, it is a vehicle for interpretation as well as for recording (see Croy (1973) for an outline of graphic processes).

As with drawing from the compound microscope, the major and initial difficulty is to obtain accurate outlines of the whole area to be portrayed; if finer details are also needed they are usually added later using a higher power. Several methods of obtaining such outlines are available in the macro range, especially for transmitted-light work. These techniques have much to commend them, for even a beginner can produce satisfactory (professional-looking) results with their aid, provided a suitable set of drawing pens is used (such as those made by Rotring). These pens must be able to provide accurate widths of line, they must be held vertically to allow them to do so, and definite controlled movement of the pen is vital; at all costs, sketchiness must be avoided in such scientific work. Making lines of consistent definite widths to suit definite structures in the original is the way emphasis is provided. These rules apply to all kinds of drawing from microscopical originals, for if a drawing becomes a sketch the reader may be deterred from considering the actual content of a picture.

In all the methods described in the following sections for making drawings, it is very desirable that the photograph is made first and is to hand during the drawing. Not only is this a guide to the amount of detail needed in the drawing, but it is easy to put the slide into an instrument the wrong way round relative to the photograph (making a mirror-image drawing); if this is done, either the drawing or the photograph would have to be redone before publication!

### 7.2.1 Inking over a photographic print

It is not difficult to make a *faint* (but still detailed) bromide print of the final size required, and then to use *waterproof Indian ink* to draw over as much detail on this as required, allow it thoroughly to dry (for some hours at least), and then bleach out the original photographic image with one of the standard formulae (Jacobson *et al.*, 1988). Either the negative of the subject may be used, or the original slide (if it is of a large specimen) may be used to make a negative print. The bromide print (which can be on RC paper or fibre-based paper) may have to be made quite large. As in all graphics work, line drawings are reduced in size for printing (usually to either 66% or 50% of the original), as this improves the printed quality considerably. Further, it is a good idea to leave quite large margins round the linework itself, to allow for the addition of lead lines and labels (usually these are printed and stuck on), and also to have a margin outside these to allow for the edges or corners being slightly damaged in handling without affecting the area to be printed (which might otherwise require redrawing).

Details can be omitted or added (the title must make this clear), and as much shading, stippling or dotting added as is needed for the desired information to be conveyed. For large areas of shading, mechanical tints are available in sheets, which can be cut out and accurately applied to particular areas; this can save a large amount of time, and also looks good in the final drawing.

### 7.2.2 Using an enlarger

Another method of making an outline of even larger sections is to put the original preparation upside down in the negative carrier of the enlarger, project it at the required size on to the baseboard, and trace around required areas with a soft (but sharp) pencil. The pencil lines are easily erased once the Indian ink drawing is *fully* dry.

### 7.2.3 Using a projection mirror or drawing tube

If a compound microscope (stereo, ordinary or specialized) was used at low power to make the macro-range record, it is usually possible to project the image in some way so that an outline can be pencilled in. An actual drawing tube (the modern and much more easily used version of the camera lucida) is attachable to most modern microscopes used with the lowest power objectives. Variable areas can be drawn using such a device, although it may be necessary to move the slide once or twice so as to cover all the required area. If a drawing tube is needed, it is necessary that provision is also made for moving the drawing board. Once the relative brightnesses of the page and the image are matched, the pencil point is superimposed on the image as seen, and it is easy to trace whatever outlines are needed.

If an actual drawing tube is not available for the particular instrument used to make the macrograph, a prism or mirror may be attachable to project an image for tracing. For example, an arm can carry quite a large (good-quality) mirror angled well above the eyepiece of a stereo microscope for this purpose, or a right-angle prism can be rigged up directly over an eyepiece; this would require the paper to be held vertically, perhaps on a wall, but this is adequate for occasional use.

### 7.2.4 Reflected-light drawing

Many of the subjects recorded by reflected light are active, as well as three-dimensional. It follows that if a drawing is needed of such a record, it is likely to have to be made from a negative or transparency. The use of an enlarger for this purpose as described in Section 7.2.2 is the best choice. (It will not matter if a negative print is made to draw around and bleach out, although a colour transparency to trace around is even better than a monochrome negative.) If details are to be added to an original from an active subject, they can be synthesized from several frames quite satisfactorily.

## 7.3 Black and white photography

Modern monochrome materials are excellent in quality and, if the usual advice to choose a film and then stick to it has been followed perhaps too rigorously by a particular photographer, some experiments with new films may be advocated. The following recommendations are based on the author's own trials with the films he has used; many others are, of course, available and those interested should try them for particular jobs. For most monochrome work in the macro range, the author uses only two films (T-Max 100 and Technical Pan); with two developers (HC-110 and PQ Universal), these give a range of six definite contrast indexes, and 98% of subjects, in both reflected and transmitted light, are accommodated by them. The aim is to provide a negative which will print on normal contrast paper; this is important, for if a negative prints only on extreme-grade paper, not only is there no leeway in producing a print with a proper range of tones but the negative itself is a poor one. A poor negative cannot produce a good print.

For macro work with reflected light, where strong contrasts can be generated, a trial should be made with a contrast index of 0.5 or 0.7. For transmitted-light work with subjects of high inherent contrast, such as darkground, a contrast index of 0.7 may also prove ideal. For stained histological slides, an index of 1.5 will usually be suitable, but if contrast filters are used an index of 1.0 may be better, and this applies also to phase contrast and DIC work. For flash photographs of living organisms an index of 2.0 will probably be needed, and for reflected-light pictures of low-contrast specimens such as polished metals an index of 2.5 may well be correct. All this is summarized in *Table 7.2*, in which the speed quoted is the starting point for calibration of the equipment with trial exposures. Contrast index is a Kodak-inspired value, similar to gamma, but which also takes into account any exposure on the toe of the characteristic curve, and as a result is more realistic in practice (see Kodak publication F-5; Anon., 1990).

Both films are available in 35 mm, roll-film and sheet-film formats. Kodak HC-110 developer is sold in two sizes and viscosities; the thinner liquid in the smaller size is easier to use. The bottles give instructions for dilution to various lettered strengths; those used in *Table 7.2* are dilutions B, D and F. Any PQ Universal developer (as used for developing bromide papers) is suitable for use with Technical Pan films, but if used with T-Max 100 it gives high fog levels and staining, and control of contrast in this way is not recommended.

In the very few cases where still higher contrast is required, an emulsion such as Agfa Ortho 25 film (actually intended for copying line drawings), developed in a PQ Universal paper developer, will be satisfactory. The emulsion is available in 35 mm, roll-film and sheet-film formats; use an initial speed of 25ASA, and process in PQ Universal 1:6 for 6 min at 20°C to obtain a contrast index of about 3.2.

When only part of a bottle of monochrome or colour developer has been used, the rest can be preserved by squirting into it a good blast of a dust-off aerosol, with the tube close to the surface of the liquid; this displaces the oxygen and minimizes later oxidation.

When processing films, the author uses continuous agitation in a rotating tube processor (the Jobo); all are treated alike and results are thus comparable between films. This is important, whatever process is used. Do NOT be tempted to exceed the stated processing temperature. Do NOT be tempted to exceed the stated processing time. What is needed to control contrast accurately is accuracy in processing. Use an acid stop bath with plenty of agitation, and fix thoroughly in a hardening rapid fixer with plenty of inversion before inspecting. After washing, which need not be unduly prolonged, add a TINY amount of rinsing agent to the final wash

**Table 7.2:** Variable contrast indexes

| Contrast index | Film | Developer at 20°C | Development time (min) | Speed (ASA) |
|---|---|---|---|---|
| 0.5 | T-Max 100 | HC-110 (B) | 7 | 80 |
| 0.7 | T-Max 100 | HC-110 (B) | 11 | 100 |
| 1.0 | Technical Pan | HC-110 (F) | 13 | 64 |
| 1.5 | Technical Pan | HC-110 (D) | 6 | 100 |
| 2.0 | Technical Pan | HC-110 (B) | 10 | 150 |
| 2.5 | Technical Pan | PQ Universal (1 : 6) | 3 | 150 |

water in the tank, shake off excess water while the film is still in the reel, and hang up to dry without squeegeeing.

## 7.3.1  UV and infrared monochrome films

Sometimes the near UV wavelengths are used in macro work, often for forensic purposes. All emulsions are sensitive to these wavelengths, and the film can be chosen for the contrast required. The source must provide plenty of the required wavelengths, which cannot be short if glass lenses are to be used. Focusing through a deep blue filter is usual to minimize differences in focus between wavelengths. Processing is normal, but exposure trials may be needed compared with using white light, since many emulsions are especially sensitive to the red end, and may appear slow to the blue in consequence.

Infrared films must be specially purchased, and the choice is limited. They are used for a few special purposes, such as penetrating chitin as well as for forensic work. In 35 mm and $4 \times 5$ inch sheet film, Kodak high-speed infrared emulsion is available; in roll film only Konica 750 nm infrared film is available, and both are more expensive than films of ordinary sensitivity. Basic exposure indexes are 64ASA for the Kodak and 25ASA for the Konica, when processed in HC-110 (B) for 7 min at 20°C. Use of a powerful tungsten–halogen source is recommended to ensure the presence of enough longer wavelengths in the illumination, and it is worth noting that fibre-optic sources have lost many of their long wavelengths before their light gets to the subject. The preparation is focused with a deep red filter in place (but the exposure is measured in white light), before a visually opaque, very deep red filter is installed for the actual exposure to cut out all shorter wavelengths. (The emulsions are also sensitive to some of these.) This allows the image to form from the infrared only, makes for a sharper result, and emphasizes the infrared effects. Calibration for exposure is of course required.

## 7.3.2  Instant films for monochrome work

Polaroid make a wide range of monochrome instant films for large-format cameras; their Type 65 has uses in the macro range, providing medium contrast and a permanent negative as well as an instant print. It requires compensation to its nominal speed at exposures exceeding 1 sec. For 35 mm cameras, using a dedicated Polaroid Autoprocessor, Polapan CT has similar uses. The use of these instant materials carries a financial penalty, but the speed of access to results may justify the outlay, especially when setting up difficult reflected-light shots.

## 7.3.3  Darkroom work in monochrome

No matter how advanced, complete and modern the equipment used to form the image in the camera, and no matter how skilled the operator, much can be lost in processing the negative and in making the print. The darkroom is often a very weak link in the photographic chain; the arrangements and equipment may be outmoded, the technique may have become sloppy, and the chemicals may well be overused. The basic division in the darkroom is between wet and dry benches. The dry benches should be rigorously kept that way; it is a matter of personal technique to wash and dry the fingers when leaving the wet bench to work at the dry, and it avoids stains and other spoiled results. The wet bench is a sink of ample size, set at a height at which the operator can lean on its edge while manipulating its contents, which avoids much backache and fatigue; the back and sides of the sink should have built-in splash guards. Much could be said of personal technique in the darkroom but it would not be peculiar to macro-range work, and it must suffice here to say that there is no substitute for a year or two spent in a well-run commercial darkroom to learn all the many tricks of the trade and to acquire a rigorous approach. (Basic details of darkroom work and design are given by Langford (1984) and Schofield (1981).)

It is well to avoid mixing chemicals in the darkroom, particularly if they are in powder form; the dust which inevitably escapes cannot all be swept up (even if an occasional attempt is made), and it WILL affect negatives and prints in due course.

Proper processing equipment is an individual choice, but the weak link is usually the enlarger – especially its lenses. Since it is kept in the dark, such equipment is rarely inspected properly for wear and tear, even if it was a good model when new. There is no point at all in buying an expensive camera and microscope, and then skimping on the enlarger and its lens. The author uses El-Nikkor lenses in Durst enlargers for all formats from 35 mm to half-plate and this has proved an unbeatable combination. Durst exposure aids are used (saving money and time) and proper safelighting is installed (i.e. it is ample in intensity and of proven safety relative to the emulsions exposed to it). In that regard, if infrared films are used, test the darkroom for infrared safety on a bright sunny day, and not in a midwinter rainstorm. Any white light used for inspecting prints should have its switch high up on the wall, set sideways. It may be marked with a small piece of luminous tape.

The proper quality of a final print is judged only after much experience. It should be seen in the light of its intended use, and if it is made for a particular printer he should see an early specimen for depth and range of tones before all the rest are made. A large number of very poor half-tones still appear in the literature; they cost just as much as good ones, and detract from the quality of the author's text. What is usually needed is fairly high contrast but without the blacks being totally dense.

Keep the enlarger and its lens surfaces (all of them) clean, by applying a dust-off aerosol frequently. A clean paper handkerchief wetted with isopropanol will clean negative carriers (and spectacles) and the like very effectively, leaving them static-free.

# 7.4 Working in colour

Matching the colour film to the colour temperature of the source is a necessary consideration, for negative as well as positive films. Elementary points, such as using neutral density filters and not a voltage control to vary the intensity of a lamp, must be taken for granted in colour work. Despite these points, working with colour transparency materials is often easier than working with monochrome, for they have the high inherent contrast needed for most macro-range work. Modern tungsten emulsions are a good match for tungsten–halogen sources (although ordinary tungsten requires filtering), as daylight is for electronic flash.

## 7.4.1 Colour transparency work

The author has tested and calibrated films for his own work from two manufacturers; others should make their own choices from the many available, taking into account that the range changes day by day in modern times, since manufacturers often produce emulsions suited to particular kinds of commercial work. For flash, Kodak Ektachrome 64 (available in 35 mm, roll and sheet films) is sharp and gives good results, with a calibration starting point of 64ASA. When more speed is needed (as in reflected-light work) Kodak Ektachrome 100 Plus (also in the same formats) has excellent colour saturation, and a calibration starting point of 100ASA. For tungsten light, Kodak Ektachrome 64T and Ektachrome 160T are fine; both are available in the same formats as those already mentioned and have calibration starting points of 64ASA and 160ASA, respectively. Fujichrome 64T is another excellent tungsten emulsion, in sheet- and roll-film sizes and 35 mm, and with a calibration starting point of 64ASA.

In processing these films the E6 process is used, or a modern modification using fewer baths. When necessary, all the above can be push-processed to double their effective speeds without noticeable loss of quality, but very careful control of temperature is vital for proper processing. The author uses Chrome Six one-shot chemicals supplied by Photo Technology Ltd in a Jobo processor (Tinsley, 1992), and obtains excellent results consistently. Colour transparencies of transmitted-light work can be evaluated very easily, by checking that the background is white and one shade of density darker than pure transparent. If transparencies must be trade processed, it may be found that a wide variation in results occurs between some trade laboratories and also within a laboratory over time. In this context, it may be worth reporting that the Agfa processing centre will accept E6 process films of any make, and the author has found their work impeccable over many years. All that is needed is to buy a prepaid mailer from a dealer and send off the 120 or 35 mm film in it by post (Agfachrome Service, see Appendix).

## 7.4.2 Colour prints from colour transparencies

Making Ilfochrome (original name Cibachrome) prints from colour transparencies is a simple matter, especially from transmitted-light macrographs (Anon., 1987). The transparency is *known* to be satisfactory from simple inspection when it is chosen for printing, by its mere appearance to the eye. The process needs very little filtration in the enlarger, beyond that specified with the particular packet of paper as the initial pack. Ilford supply suitable packs of chemicals, and the process is not too demanding. The result is also easy to evaluate (but the print must be dry): simple inspection shows at once whether or not the background is white and one shade darker than pure white. The author has a daylight-blue spotlamp in a ceiling-mounted fitting (with the switch on it) especially for evaluating such prints in uniform conditions. Transparency materials can be used similarly to make very large pictures for back-lighting, and the prints are much more lightfast than other colour prints. If Ilfochrome prints of similar subjects are to be made commercially, there is no argument possible on delivery as to their correctness, of course!

## 7.4.3 Colour negative films

Many photographers use colour negative film such as Kodak Gold 200 for their casual holiday snaps, and the same can be applied to the macro range, although it is unusual. All colour negative films should be generously exposed in all circumstances, by setting the camera half a stop slower than the nominal speed of the film. In macro work, of course, proper calibration will be carried out to arrive at a definite result. If a tungsten source is used with an ordinary colour negative film, a daylight-blue correcting filter should be interposed, as it will make selecting the final printing pack very much easier. If this type of work is done often, a film balanced for longer exposures should be used; Fujicolour 160L is suitable in the author's experience. This is in addition to any considerations of colour temperature; long exposures with ordinary films (which are made for short exposures) may result in the characteristic curves crossing, making it impossible to print them with proper colour balance.

Printing colour negative films is slightly more difficult than printing positive films in that the choice of the filter pack and exposure time is less obvious. It can, however, be carried out very successfully using the Photocolor FP two-bath kits supplied by Photo Technology Ltd, which process both C41 and RA4 materials very successfully. Some aid to negative evaluation is desirable for speed and economy; the author uses Durst instruments, but many other makes are available.

## 7.4.4 Infrared colour films

Kodak produce a 35 mm infrared colour film, in 36 exposure cassettes, which can be used occasionally in the macro range, especially in forensic work. The emulsion is also available to order as Aerochrome Infrared Type 2443 (as 70 mm perforated film, and intended for aerial photography, especially in detecting camouflage). The 35 mm film is called Ektachrome Infrared Film Type 2236. It is, unfortunately, processed in E4 chemicals, which are rarely called for, and for which it is difficult to find a commercial processor (although a kit called Speedibrews E-4 can be obtained from Silver Print Ltd, see Appendix). The film produces 'false-colour' results, having an infrared-sensitive, cyan-image-forming layer instead of the usual blue-sensitive layer. There is no yellow filter layer in this daylight-balanced film, and thus a yellow filter (Kodak Wratten Type 12 or equivalent) must be used over the taking lens. It has about twice the effective speed of Kodak high-speed infrared film, but equipment and lighting must be calibrated not only for speed but also to determine the colour translation of the particular subjects being recorded. It is essential to store this film at no higher a temperature than $-20°C$ to avoid loss of infrared sensitivity.

As examples of colour translation, healthy deciduous green leaves appear red while diseased leaves appear greenish-blue; venous blood appears red–brown while arterial blood appears green–brown; unstained bacteria are reddish; yellow tends to appear as blue; green often appears as magenta; and black dyes often appear as dark red. The film produces interesting results that are obtainable in no other way.

### 7.4.5 Instant films for colour work

Polaroid supply a number of colour print instant films, including Polacolor 64 Tungsten which may be of occasional interest in macro-range work, as it gives rich and saturated colours with exposures in the range 2–8 sec in sheet-film sizes. Their Polachrome CS and HC films are of interest as quick-access 35 mm reversal films (daylight-balanced), intended specifically for projection, and thus valuable for preparing lecture material in small quantities and at short notice.

### 7.4.6 Recording motion. 1: analogue movie films

The application of the cine camera to macro-range work is far from obsolete. Sequences for natural history television programmes, for example, are still recorded on motion-picture film, and one specialist in the macro range even uses IMAX cameras (taking 70 mm film sideways, at breathtaking expense) fitted with tubes and macro lenses for his superb results. Any sequence of living or other mobile things requires such work, and the quality and cost still compares favourably with broadcast-quality closed-circuit television (CCTV) recording. The easy availability of slow-motion and time-lapse techniques with cine is a further powerful argument in its favour. Most of the various techniques of the lighting cameraman are available in the macro range, and cannot be described here

(Baddeley, 1979; Fielding, 1985; Reisz and Millar, 1994; Souto, 1984; Spottiswoode *et al.*, 1969), but it is easy enough to couple a movie camera with macro-range apparatus. For occasional use where standards need not be too high in quality, any ordinary 16 mm or even 8 mm camera can be used with its (fixed) lens in apposition to the end of the optics of the stereomicroscope or Makroskop; alignment is by inspection (preferably of a test target) through the viewfinder. Better results are obtained using more sophisticated macro equipment and more serious cameras, of 16 mm or even 35 mm format, with the usual C mount for its lenses; no lens is used, of course, and alignment can be better obtained, although a relay lens may be needed to place the image in the film plane. Use of really heavy stands is an initial requirement, and rigorous setting up helps to avoid a large wastage of the resources inherent in motion-picture filming. A good range of film stock is available, covering most requirements, and many processing houses provide excellent service. Much of the success of motion-picture work resides in the final editing, and a ratio of 10:1 between film footage shot and that finally used is good. Some modification of the final image is possible, but tedious, and the medium can be essentially straight-forward for scientific recording.

### 7.4.7 Recording motion. 2: analogue video recording

The coupling of ordinary video cameras to macro-range apparatus from the 1950s onwards had immediate advantages for viewing the image. The picture was produced in real time, could have its contrast dramatically increased, could be generated from very low light levels, and could give results from wavelengths normally invisible. With the advent of increasingly inexpensive video cassette recorders and new types of cameras (by the 1980s), colour as well as monochrome images could be stored easily and cheaply. There is no doubt that the application of CCTV to recording images generated by the microscopy of active subjects has made the interpretation of such subjects much easier, and the almost universal availability of domestic camcorders now allows even the beginner to record his observations more easily than ever before (the standard basic text is Inoué, 1986; a basic introduction to modern video is provided by Cheshire, 1990).

For fixed-lens models (which may be very sophisticated in other ways), and using a stereomicroscope or a Makroskop, all that is needed is to suspend the camera over the output tube of the instrument which is fitted with a large-diameter projection lens (possibly from a slide projector) in an extension tube, instead of the usual eyepiece. The length of this extension tube is that needed to project the primary image to infinity, as determined by experiment. The image is adjusted visually, the ordinary eyepiece removed, and the projection eyepiece inserted. The camera, with its zoom lens set to infinity at its longest focus, is arranged to leave an initial gap of about 20 mm between its front and the projection lens; this gap is then adjusted to focus the image by checking the monitor. The zoom settings can then be used to place more or less of the image circle on the sensor, thus varying the apparent magnification (Thomson, 1991).

For video cameras fitted with a C mount and used with a stereomicroscope or the like, its lens is removed and a normal projection eyepiece is used (possibly with a relay lens) to focus the image on the sensor in the usual way. The camera can also be fitted at the film plane of, say, a long-bellows camera; less extension than usual will be needed, of course, as the image area is small. The author has modified a darkslide to carry a C-mount adapter; this fits on to the back of the 4 × 5 inch camera to carry the video camera. Alternatively, such an adapter can be fitted to a 35 mm bellows or extension tube direct, with a mount for the macro lens at the other end; this makes a very compact unit, which can even be used hand-held if need be (*Figure 7.1*).

Modern equipment provides quite high-quality colour images, and even 3 h recording tapes are cheap to buy and reuseable. For simple recording of active subjects with basic contrast enhancement and colour-balance modification, such equipment is hard to beat, and not impossibly expensive for occasional use even by the amateur.

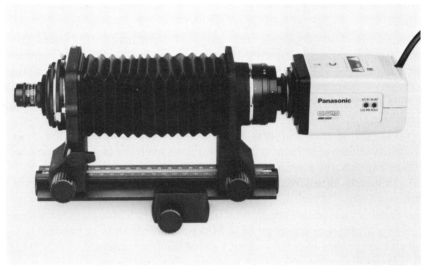

**Figure 7.1:** CCTV unit ready for use.
The bellows unit carries an adapter at its lens end, taking any RMS-threaded macro lens. An adapter at the other end has a C mount, to take a small CCD CCTV camera. A wide range of magnifications is possible with such a unit. It should be remembered that such a camera can work in very low light levels and auxiliary lighting may not be needed, although a reflector is often useful. Instant viewing of results is the norm, and instant replay of a sequence is very easy. Hand-holding at magnifications of even × 5 or ×10 is possible, with suitable stance, and manipulation of the results of digital recordings (e.g. to clean up the background) is easy.

# 7.5 Digital recording for image modification

The advent of equipment for digitizing images, however generated, allows such stored images to be manipulated (processed and analysed) and transmitted in astonishing ways. A note of some of the possibilities is all that can be included in the present volume, with a word of caution added (see Larish (1991) for a survey of digital imaging). Particular items of equipment are not specified, as new ones are introduced on an almost weekly basis, and are equally rapidly superseded.

Existing analogue macro images or others, transparencies or prints, colour or monochrome, line or half-tone, can be scanned into electronic digitized storage, or analogue images can be scanned as generated, say in macro-range equipment of whatever kind. In either case, a continuously varying analogue input is converted into discrete steps, of binary form (to be stored as individual bits in a computer) by sampling it at varying intervals. The shorter the intervals, the more accurate is (the higher the quality of) the sampling. Equipment for amateur-quality digitally stored picture-making is already a consumer product. The newer CCD-type chips used even in small modern TV cameras produce a digital output in pixel form. Images can be sent to a monitor, or stored on WORM (write once, read many) optical discs.

Equipment for high-quality scanning or digitizing is still expensive, but rapidly becoming less so; it is likely to be ubiquitous in professional photography by the end of the decade. Equipment for direct digitizing in-camera, in large and thus high-quality formats such as $4 \times 5$ inch, is now available; although it is currently very expensive, it is likely to become much less so. Setting-up such a camera with its rather bulky back is just the same as with a sheet of film, but as the scanning device must traverse the image (taking about a minute), this kind of capture is limited to static subjects. It also produces a file of about 100 megabytes.

The stored image is a series of points, picture-elements or pixels, shown on screen as a tiny square filled with one hue of colour or shade of grey. Once captured in this way, the picture can be copied electronically with no loss of quality, or transferred instantly like a telephone message along wire or by satellite. More to the point, it can be enhanced or cleaned up or modified, without detection, until it resembles the original only slightly or not at all. All this is accomplished at the computer screen, and needs skill and purpose on the part of the operator; in a non-scientific situation, it can require artistic ability of a high order to produce absolutely stunning images, perhaps seamlessly put together from several sources. Once the desired image is obtained, it is simply output to a suitable printer.

In the scientific context, it has long been the case that stored digitized images can be analysed to extract data rapidly and accurately; image analysis is a very important and developing area of data manipulation, with established procedures (Bradbury, 1987; Russ, 1990). Now that image manipulation is also becoming established, with processing platforms possessing very powerful software, and hard-copy output devices producing high-quality results, those producing scientific photographs are going to have to declare exactly to what extent the final image has been manipulated – merely reducing signal-to-noise ratio, enhancing colour or rather more. The range of printers is now large, and good quality is obtained easily and cheaply from developed thermal wax and inkjet printers, while dye sublimation prints can be made in minutes in sizes as large as A0 in stunning quality.

These means of dealing with images produced using macro-range apparatus are very powerful indeed in their possibilities and implications, and are likely to become widespread quite rapidly.

# References

**Anon.** (1987) *Ilford Cibachrome-A.* Ilford, London.

**Anon.** (1990) *Kodak Professional Black-and-White Films.* Kodak publication F-5, Rochester.

**Baddeley WH.** (1979) *The Technique of Documentary Film Production.* Focal Press, London.

**Bradbury S.** (1987) Processing and analysis of the microscope image. *Quekett J. Microsc.* **36**, 23–39.

**Cheshire D.** (1990) *The Complete Book of Video.* Dorling Kindersely, London.

**Croy P.** (1973) *Graphic Design and Reproduction Techniques* (2nd Edn). Focal Press, London.

**Fielding R.** (1985) *The Technique of Special Effects Cinematography* (4th Edn). Focal Press, London.

**Inoué S.** (1986) *Video Microscopy.* Plenum Press, New York.

**Jacobson RE, Ray SF, Attridge GG.** (1988) *The Manual of Photography* (8th Edn). Focal Press, London.

**Langford M.** (1984) *The Darkroom Handbook* (2nd Edn). Ebury Press, London.

**Langford M.** (1986) *Basic Photography* (5th Edn). Focal Press, London.

**Langford M.** (1989) *Advanced Photography.* Focal Press, London.

**Larish J.** (1992) *Digital Photography: Pictures of Tomorrow.* Micro Publishing Press, Torrance.

**Morton RA. (ed.)** (1984) *Photography for the Scientist* (2nd Edn). Academic Press, London.

**Ray SF.** (1983) *Camera Systems.* Focal Press, London.

**Ray SF.** (1994) *Applied Photographic Optics* (2nd Edn). Focal Press, London.

**Reisz K, Millar G.** (1994) *The Technique of Film Editing.* Focal Press, London.

**Russ JC.** (1990) *Computer-assisted Microscopy.* Plenum Press, New York.

**Schofield J. (ed.)** (1981) *The Darkroom Book.* Newnes, Feltham.

**Souto HMR.** (1984) *The Technique of the Motion Picture Camera.* Focal Press, London.

**Spottiswoode R. (ed.).** (1969) *The Focal Encyclopaedia of Film and Television Techniques.* Focal Press, London.

**Stroebel L, Compton J, Current I, Zakia R.** (1990) *Basic Photographic Materials and Processes.* Focal Press, London.

**Thomson DJ.** (1991) Video microscopy using a TV camera fitted with a zoom lens. *Microscopy Bulletin, the Newsletter of the Quekett Microscopical Club* **17**, 12–13.

**Tinsley J.** (1992) *The Rotary Processor Manual.* R Morgan, Chislehurst.

# Appendix
## Manufacturers and suppliers

Agfachrome Service, PO Box 32, Bury, Lancs BL9 0AD, UK.

Camera Bellows, Lee Filters, Central Way, Walworth Industrial Estate, Andover, Hants SP10 5AN, UK.

Electromail, PO Box 33, Corby, Northants NN17 9EL, UK.

Fostec Inc., 62 Columbus Street, Auburn, NY 13021–0275, USA. Manufacturers of the Fostec Darkfield Illuminator P/N 8640, with adapters to fit Olympus BH2, Nikon Labphot and Zeiss Axioskop substages. This will illuminate a darkground field of up to diameter 25 mm at a working distance of 0–10 mm.

Fotogerätebau K. Müller, PO Box 1744, D-8940, Memmingen, Germany. Manufacturers of the Novoflex 'Macrolight Plus', a fibre-optic lamphousing with triple lightguides and provision for attaching the flash unit of one's choice.

Graticules Ltd, Morley Road, Tonbridge, Kent TN9 1RN, UK. Manufacturers of the England finder.

Irvine Optical Corporation, 1713 West Magnolia Road, Burbank, CA 91506, USA. Suppliers of the Dynaphot.

H. Makowsky, Cologne, Germany.

Micro Video Instruments Inc., 11 Robbie Road, PO Box 518, Avon, MA 02322, USA. Suppliers of the Darklite Illuminator.

Photo Technology Ltd, Potters Bar, Herts EN6 3JN, UK.

Prior Scientific Instruments Ltd, Unit 4, Wilbraham Road, Fulbourn, Cambridge CB1 5ET, UK.

Questar Corporation, RD1, New Hope, PA 18938, USA.

RS Components, PO Box 99, Corby, Northants NN17 9RS, UK. RS products are available through Electromail (see above) a mail order company trading on a cash-with-order or credit card basis in the UK.

Silver Print Ltd, 12 Valentine Place, London SE1 5QH, UK. Suppliers of Speedibrews E-4. (Processing of E-4 films is offered by Argentum, 1 Wimpole Street, London W1M 8AE, UK.)

SRB Film Service, 286 Leagrave Road, Luton, Beds LU3 1RB, UK. Manufacture and supply modestly priced adapter rings of all kinds. Also manufacture individual components to order.

# Index

# OTHER MICROSCOPY HANDBOOKS

Confocal Laser Scanning
Microscopy
C. Sheppard & D. Shotton

Food Microscopy
O. Flint

Enzyme Histochemistry
A Laboratory Manual of Current
Methods
C. J. F. van Noorden &
W. M. Frederiks

The Role of Microscopy in
Semiconductor Failure Analysis
B. P. Richards & P. K. Footner

Qualitative Polarized-Light
Microscopy
P. C. Robinson & S. Bradbury

The Preparation of Thin
Sections of Rocks, Minerals
and Ceramics
D. W. Humphries

Introduction to Crystallography
Revised Edition
C. Hammond

Basic Measurement Techniques
for Light Microscopy
S. Bradbury

An Introduction to Surface
Analysis Electron Spectroscopy
J. F. Watts

Cryopreparation of Thin
Biological Specimens for
Electron Microscopy
Methods and Applications
N. Roos & A. J. Morgan

The Operation of Transmission
and Scanning Electron
Microscopes
D. Chescoe & P. J. Goodhew

Autoradiography
A Comprehensive Overview
J. R. J. Baker

RMS Dictionary of Light
Microscopy
Compiled by the Nomenclature
Committee of the RMS

An Introduction to the Optical
Microscope
Revised Edition
S. Bradbury

Colloidal Gold
A New Perspective for Cytochemical
Marking
J. E. Beesley

Light-Element Analysis in the
Transmission Electron
Microscope
WEDX and EELS
P. M. Budd & P. J. Goodhew

An Introduction to Scanning
Acoustic Microscopy
A. Briggs

An Introduction to
Immunocytochemistry
Current Techniques and Problems
Revised Edition
J. M. Polak & S. van Noorden

Maintaining and Monitoring the
Transmission Electron
Microscope
S. K. Chapman

X-Ray Microanalysis in Electron
Microscopy for Biologists
A. J. Morgan

Lipid Histochemistry
O. Bayliss High

# Biological Microtechnique

**J. Sanderson**
Sir William Dunn School of Pathology, Oxford, UK

Although many significant advances have been made in biological specimen preparation during the past 20 years no new practical guide to the techniques has been published in this time. As a result of the recent resurgence of interest in light microscopy, particularly confocal techniques, this new, up-to-date book will benefit both novices and experienced microscopists seeking to extend their repertoire of techniques.

A poorly-prepared specimen inevitably leads to unreliable results. This new book therefore describes both new and classical methods of slide-making in an easy-to-read, easy-to-understand format. It contains a wealth of practical detail which will provide a firm grounding in preparative methods for light microscopy.

## Contents

Fixation; Tissue processing; Microtomy; Other preparative methods; Staining and dyeing; Finishing the preparation. Appendices: safety; removing dyestains; restaining faded sections; restoring tissues; cleaning glassware; physiological solutions; saturation.

## Of interest to:

Junior researchers, laboratory technicians, skilled amateur microscopists, undergraduates, school science teachers and students.

Paperback; 240 pages; 1-872748-42-2; 1994

# Flow Cytometry

**M.G. Ormerod**
Scientific Consultant, Reigate, Surrey, UK

Flow cytometry is a specialised form of microscopy for measuring the properties of single cells. Flow cytometers are becoming widely used in clinical and research laboratories and there is an increasing need for non-specialists to have an understanding of this technology. *Flow Cytometry* is a practical guide to the instrumentation and the application of this method in mammalian cell biology. The book is easy to read and contains sufficient information and references to allow the reader to pursue any particular application in greater depth. It covers the routine applications of flow cytometry and introduces the reader to the more recent applications of this exciting technology.

## Contents

What is flow cytometry; Instrumentation; Fluorescence; Immunofluorescence; Analysis of DNA; Study of cell proliferation and death; Other applications. *Appendices:* Glossary; Suppliers; Learned societies.

## Of interest to:

Postgraduates, clinicians, researchers, technicians and all first-time users.

Paperback; 88 pages;  1-872748-39-2; 1994

ALSO AVAILABLE FROM BIOS SCIENTIFIC PUBLISHERS LTD

# Food Microscopy

**O. Flint**
University of Leeds, Leeds, UK

A practical guide to using optical microscopy for examining the microstructure of food products and obtaining information to complement chemical and physical analyses. The book covers a range of practical techniques with the emphasis on rapid methods and includes sufficient theoretical background information to understand the mechanisms involved. After reading this book, a microscopist should be able to select and modify the techniques to make them suitable for individual food products.

## Contents

Introduction; Choice of equipment; Preparation of food for the stereomicroscope; Simple preparation techniques for the compound microscope; Use of the food cryostat in food microscopy; Contrast techniques for food constituents; Fat in food; Food starches; Vegetable proteins; The Howard mould count of Tomato products; Food gums; Food emulsions.

## Of interest to:

Undergraduates, postgraduates and researchers in food science; industrial food scientists.

Paperback; 144 pages; 1-872748-04-X; 1994

# In Situ Hybridization

**A.R. Leitch, T. Schwarzacher, D. Jackson & I.J. Leitch**
respectively Queen Mary and Westfield College, London, UK; John Innes
Research Centre, Norwich, UK; USDA, Plant Gene Expression Center,
Albany, California, USA; and Royal Botanic Gardens, Kew, UK

*In situ* hybridization is a powerful link beween cellular and molecular biology.
This practical guide provides a comprehensive description of *in situ*
hybridization, from background information to detailed methodology and
practical applications.

The book's clarity of approach and up-to-date coverage of methods and
troubleshooting makes it the ideal introduction for all first-time users and a
valuable companion for experienced researchers.

## Contents

Introduction; Nucleic acid sequences located *in situ*; The material; Nucleic
acid probes, labels and labelling methods; Denaturation, hybridization and
washing; Detection of the *in situ* hybridization sites; Imaging systems and the
analysis of signal; The *in situ* hybridization schedule (including
troubleshooting); The future of *in situ* hybridization. Appendix: Suppliers of
reagents and *in situ* hybridization kits; Buffers.

## Of interest to:

Advanced undergraduates and postgraduate students of molecular biology,
cell biology and genetics.

Paperback; 128 pages;  1-872748-48-1; 1994

# ORDERING DETAILS

**Main address for orders**

**BIOS Scientific Publishers Ltd**
**St Thomas House, Becket Street,**
**Oxford OX1 1SJ, UK**
**Tel: +44 1865 726286**
**Fax: +44 1865 246823**

**Australia and New Zealand**
DA Information Services
648 Whitehorse Road, Mitcham, Victoria 3132, Australia
Tel: (03) 873 4411
Fax: (03) 873 5679

**India**
Viva Books Private Ltd
4346/4C Ansari Road, New Delhi 110 002, India
Tel: 11 3283121
Fax: 11 3267224

**Singapore and South East Asia**
(Brunei, Hong Kong, Indonesia, Korea, Malaysia, the Philippines,
Singapore, Taiwan, and Thailand)
Toppan Company (S) PTE Ltd
38 Liu Fang Road, Jurong, Singapore 2262
Tel: (265) 6666
Fax: (261) 7875

**USA and Canada**
Books International Inc
PO Box 605, Herndon, VA 22070, USA
Tel: (703) 435 7064
Fax: (703) 689 0660

Payment can be made by cheque or credit card (Visa/Mastercard, quoting number and expiry date). Alternatively, a *pro forma* invoice can be sent.

Prepaid orders must include £2.50/US$5.00 to cover postage and packing for one item and £1.25/US$2.50 for each additional item.